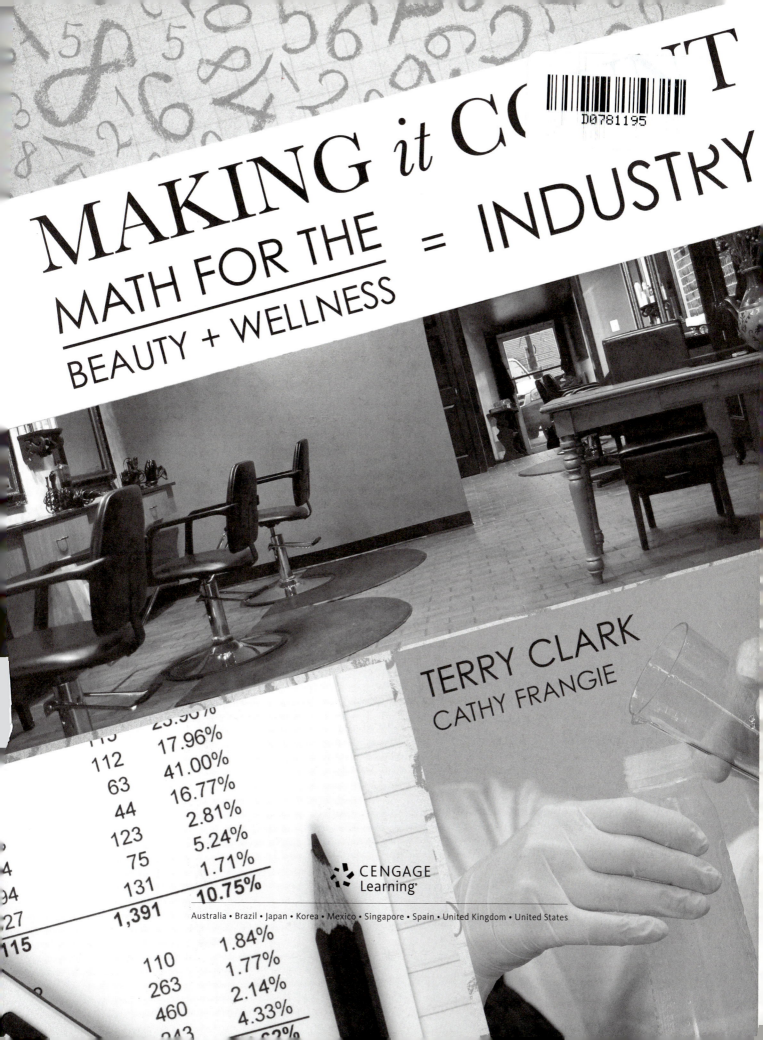

Making it Count: Math for the Beauty and Wellness Industry
Authors: Terry Freeman Clark and Catherine M. Frangie
Contributor: John Halal

Vice President, Milady & Learning Solutions Strategy, Professional: Dawn Gerrain

Director of Content & Business Development, Milady: Sandra Bruce

Senior Acquisitions Editor: Martine Edwards

Product Manager: Maria Moffre-Barnes

Editorial Assistant: Sarah Prediletto

Director, Marketing & Training: Gerard McAvey

Marketing Manager: Matthew McGuire

Senior Production Director: Wendy Troeger

Production Manager: Sherondra Thedford

Senior Content Project Manager: Stacey Lamodi

Senior Art Director: Benj Gleeksman

Cover image: Top: © DP Photography/www. Shutterstock.com; Bottom (left to right): © iStockphoto/Traveling Light; © iStockphoto/Pashabo; © Milady, a part of Cengage Learning

For product information and technology assistance, contact us at
Cengage Learning Customer & Sales Support, 1-800-354-9706

For permission to use material from this text or product, submit all requests online at **www.cengage.com/permissions**.
Further permissions questions can be e-mailed to
permissionrequest@cengage.com.

Library of Congress Control Number: 2012936030

ISBN-13: 978-1-111-64144-3

ISBN-10: 1-111-64144-7

Milady
5 Maxwell Drive
Clifton Park, NY 12065-2919
USA

Cengage Learning is a leading provider of customized learning solutions with office locations around the globe, including Singapore, the United Kingdom, Australia, Mexico, Brazil, and Japan. Locate your local office at:
international.cengage.com/region

Cengage Learning products are represented in Canada by Nelson Education, Ltd.

For your lifelong learning solutions, visit **milady.cengage.com**

Purchase any of our products at your local college store or at our preferred online store **www.cengagebrain.com**

Visit our corporate website at **cengage.com**

Notice to the Reader

Publisher does not warrant or guarantee any of the products described herein or perform any independent analysis in connection with any of the product information contained herein. Publisher does not assume, and expressly disclaims, any obligation to obtain and include information other than that provided to it by the manufacturer. The reader is expressly warned to consider and adopt all safety precautions that might be indicated by the activities described herein and to avoid all potential hazards. By following the instructions contained herein, the reader willingly assumes all risks in connection with such instructions. The publisher makes no representations or warranties of any kind, including but not limited to, the warranties of fitness for particular purpose or merchantability, nor are any such representations implied with respect to the material set forth herein, and the publisher takes no responsibility with respect to such material. The publisher shall not be liable for any special, consequential, or exemplary damages resulting, in whole or part, from the readers' use of, or reliance upon, this material.

Printed in the United States of America
1 2 3 4 5 6 7 17 16 15 14 13 12

Table of Contents

PREFACE

WHY MATH IS YOUR FRIEND!

HAVE YOU EVER THOUGHT OR SAID, "I BECAME A cosmetologist/nail tech/esthetician/massage therapist so I *wouldn't* have to do math"?

You know what's really funny about that? As a cosmetologist, nail tech, esthetician, or massage therapist, you actually "do math" all day long—you just don't realize it!

When you take a $\frac{1}{2}$-inch parting for that haircut, you're doing math! When you figure out how much a 15% tip would be on a $35 nail service, you're doing math! And when you squeeze haircolor out of a tube and add developer to it—guess what? You're doing math!

In this book, you're going to learn a little bit more about mathematics—not because you want to be a math scholar, but because it will help you to perform your work and services in the beauty and wellness field better. You will explore mathematics as it applies to beauty salons, spas, barber shops, nail salons, and massage therapy. You will uncover the rules and learn how to speak the language of mathematics, and you will learn how to solve essential math problems that will help you master the business side of beauty.

By the time you've completed your study of this text, you will know which mathematical operations are best to use and when to use them; you'll be able to easily read math problems and determine solutions; you'll be able to forecast monies, figure out your paycheck, schedule your services more efficiently, and plan for your future. In the later chapters, you'll learn how to read a Profit and Loss statement and how to figure out interest rates; you'll be an expert at creating and monitoring budgets, managing your salon or spa's inventory, and pricing your products and services so that they are profitable.

Once you know how to do it, I guarantee you won't be able to stop—you'll actually enjoy doing math, and you will feel great because you will be in control of your finances, your business, and your financial future instead of them controlling you.

Throughout this book, you will read stories and be given problems to solve that are identical to the types of situations you'll find yourself in every day. You'll get the opportunity to practice solving these problems, and you'll even create little shortcuts for yourself that will prove handy in your everyday life.

We're about to begin a fun and interesting journey—one that will provide you with an unending stream of benefits—so, let's get started!

Terry Freeman Clark
Catherine M. Frangie

ABOUT THE AUTHORS

Terry Freeman Clark

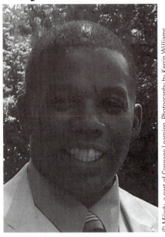

© Milady, a part of Cengage Learning. Photography by Kerrin Williams.

Terry Freeman Clark is currently the Associate Course Director and Professor of Math at Full Sail University located in Winter Park, Florida. In addition, he is an adjunct Math instructor for Columbia College and Strayer University. Terry holds a Master of Science in Mathematics Education from Nova Southeastern University and is working towards his doctorate.

Terry's talent for math education has given him the opportunity to instruct to a broad range of audiences and difficulty levels. Through his 11-year career he has instructed a variety of topics including the areas of statistics, college algebra, finite math, survey of mathematics, mathematics for elementary school teachers, middles school math, college math, and online math.

Catherine M. Frangie

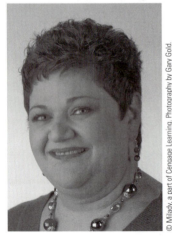

© Milady, a part of Cengage Learning. Photography by Gary Gold.

Catherine M. Frangie has been a dedicated and passionate beauty professional since 1982 when she first began her career as a licensed cosmetologist, salon owner, and beauty school instructor. Since then, Catherine has held prominent and dynamic positions throughout many facets of the professional beauty industry, including Marketing, Communications and Education Vice President for a leading product company; Communications Director; Trade Magazine Publisher; and Textbook Editor and Author.

Catherine has addressed her beauty colleagues numerous times as a guest lecturer at the International Beauty Show in New York City and in other national venues. She has personally authored more than 125 feature length trade and consumer magazine articles and several books on beauty trends, fashion, and the business of the professional salon. In 1990, Catherine was honored to be named *A Beauty Industry Role Model* by the Cosmetology Advancement Foundation (CAF) and to participate in their mentor program. Catherine holds a graduate degree in communications as well as undergraduate degrees in marketing and advertising.

In her capacity as Vice President of Marketing and Communications for Joico Laboratories, Catherine was a member of the company's Executive Team and was instrumental in creating the company's strategic vision and in directing the company to achieve its goals. During her tenure, she was responsible for more than 18 new product launches across all product categories, re-imaging campaigns for two prominent product lines, and the launch of Joico's most successful line extension ever, The K-Pak Collection.

For 11 years as Vice President of Milady Publishing Company, the leading publisher of cosmetology-related educational materials in the world, Catherine lent her vision to revamping the company's line of textbooks and to introducing their first series of educational videos. In 1993, she led Milady into the professional realm with the launch of SalonOvations Publishing, the company's salon education division. Just one year later Catherine achieved another milestone when she founded and launched *SalonOvations Magazine*, a trade publication for beauty professionals, which quickly won audience favor and grew to become the Official Publication of the National Cosmetology Association. Throughout her tenure at Milady, Catherine was the company's international spokesperson.

Catherine's experiences and successes have given her a well-deserved reputation as an industry expert on a myriad of topics ranging from marketing and communications to education and curriculum development. In 2001, she founded **Frangie**Consulting, a very unique marketing, communications and publishing firm which offers innovative strategies for managing business objectives, creating high-performing teams, and successfully achieving goals. In addition, Catherine's work has earned her seven ABBIES Awards, including two Gold ABBIES.

CHAPTER 1

Mathematical Basics

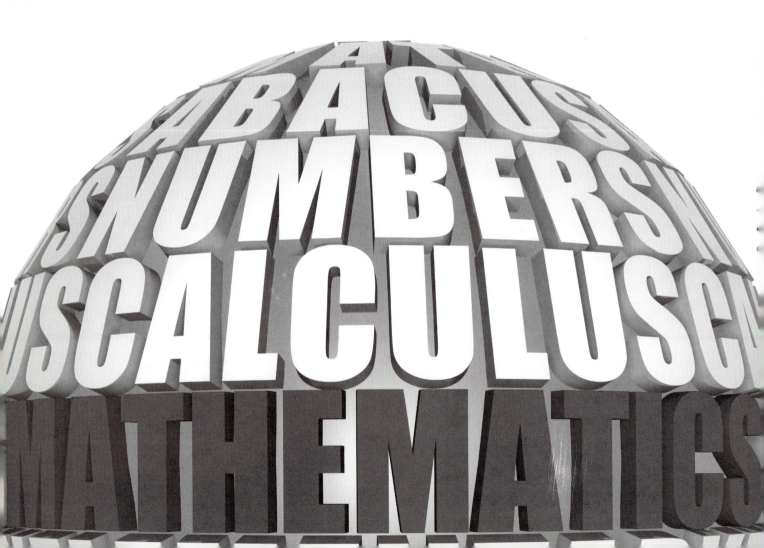

LEARNING OBJECTIVES

After completing this chapter, you will be able to:

1. Name and recognize each of the four mathematical operations used in problem-solving.

2. Identify key words within a problem that provide guidance as to which mathematical operation to use.

3. Perform addition, subtraction, multiplication, and division, and recognize their relevance to a career in the beauty and wellness industry.

4. Understand what an opposite number is and how it is used.

5. Identify and use the associative property.

6. Identify and use the commutative property.

7. Identify and use the distributive property.

8. Identify and use the identity property.

9. Identify and use the inverse property.

KEY TERMS

- addends
- addition
- associative property
- commutative property
- difference
- distributive property
- dividend
- division
- divisor
- equation
- factors
- identity property
- inverse property
- mathematical operations
- mathematical properties
- mathematics
- minuend
- multiplication
- order of operations
- product
- quotient
- subtraction
- subtrahend
- sum

MOST PROFESSIONALS SELECT A CAREER IN THE BEAUTY BUSINESS BECAUSE they enjoy using their artistic abilities to help others look and feel their best. Beauty professionals are generally good-hearted, vivacious, and hard-working people who also *want* and *need* to earn a living doing what they love. That is why it is so important to remember that the beauty business involves more than just beauty—it is also a business, and it requires that sound

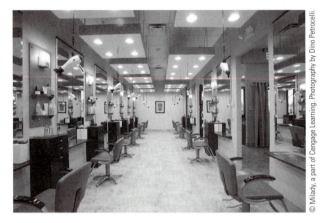

© Milady, a part of Cengage Learning. Photography by Dino Petrocelli.

business principles and management be employed so that professionals can continue to do what they love, help their clients, and earn a comfortable living as well.

Mastering mathematical basics—operations and properties—is essential to help a business be profitable so that it can *stay* in business. **Mathematical operations** are tasks that are performed between two or more numbers or groups of numbers. **Mathematical properties** are the rules or characteristics that always exist for a particular mathematical operation.

MATHEMATICAL OPERATIONS

So what is mathematics, anyway? **Mathematics** is a universal language that is expressed with numbers, graphs, shapes, symbols, and signs of operations. It is also the study of patterns. A pattern is something that occurs repeatedly until the observer is able to predict what will occur next. An **equation** is the format mathematics uses to communicate its meaning. For example, $4 + 3 = 7$ is an equation.

There are four basic mathematic operations: addition, subtraction, multiplication, and division. They are called operations because when they are placed between two numbers, they require certain tasks to be performed, such as increasing or decreasing the first number or value by the second number or value.

Addition

Addition is the *combining* of two or more groups of the same objects. The numbers that are being added are called the **addends**, and the answer that they create is called the **sum**.

An example of this concept is $6 + 4 = 10$. In this example, the *6* and *4* are the *addends* and the *10* is the *sum*. The symbol for addition is the + (plus) sign. The addition symbol requires that the first number be increased by the second number:

6	haircuts (addend)
+ 4	haircolor services (addend)
= 10	services performed in a day (sum)

WORD CLUE   Any time we are asked for a *total* we have to add. There are several words used in problems that indicate that we need to add: *all*, *total*, *increase* or *increased*, and *sum*.

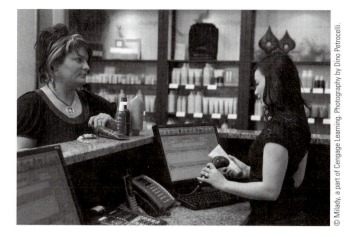

Converting Word Problems into Equations

Every story or word problem uses certain words or language to express and clue you in to the operation that must be used to solve it.

Take a look at the following example: *Mary purchased 3 items. The first cost $252, the second cost $315, and the third cost $168. How much did Mary have to pay for* **all three** *items?*

The clue words in this problem are **all three**. To convert this problem from words to numbers, you would do the following: Add $252, $315, and $168, for a total of $735.

In numbers it would look like this:

$$\begin{array}{r} \$252 \\ + \$315 \\ + \$168 \\ \hline = \$735 \end{array}$$

As you continue to learn about mathematical operations, you will be given key words to be aware of in a word problem that will help you determine the correct operation to use to solve the problem.

1-1 LET ME TRY

Note: The answer key to the LET ME TRY exercises is found at the back of the book.

Read the questions below and determine how to solve them before reading the answer—are your conclusions correct?

1. Talia ordered 6 tubes of haircolor on Monday and 4 tubes of haircolor on Friday. How many tubes of haircolor did she order in total?

2. Jason purchased 3 items. The first cost $312, the second cost $289, and the third cost $154. How much did he have to pay for all three items?

Subtraction

Subtraction is the *reducing* of two or more groups of the same objects. The number that is being reduced is called the **minuend**, and the number that is being subtracted is called the **subtrahend**. The answer that the minuend and the subtrahend create is called the **difference**.

An example of this concept is $10 - 8 = 2$. The *10* is called the *minuend*, the *8* is called the *subtrahend*, and the *2* is called the *difference*. The symbol for subtraction is the − (minus) sign. The subtraction symbol requires that the first number be decreased by the second number:

$$
\begin{array}{rl}
10 & \text{bottles of shampoo available for sale (\textbf{minuend})} \\
-8 & \text{the number of bottles of shampoo sold (\textbf{subtrahend})} \\
\hline
=2 & \text{the number of bottles of shampoo still on the retail shelf (\textbf{difference})}
\end{array}
$$

Anytime we are asked for the *difference*, we have to subtract. Other words that clue us to subtract are *change*, *less than*, *decreased*, and *difference*.

1–2 LET ME TRY

Read the questions below and determine how to solve them before reading the answer—are your conclusions correct?

1. A bottle of hair conditioner costs $6, and Maria paid the clerk with a $10 bill. How much change should Maria receive?

2. Joy charged Brenda $85 for a massage, and Brenda paid Joy with a $100 bill. How much money should be returned to Brenda?

Multiplication

Multiplication is the *combining* of one or more sets of numbers. The numbers that are being multiplied are called the **factors**, and the answer that is created is called the **product**. An example of this concept is $4 \times 7 = 28$; the *4* and *7* are called the *factors* and the *28* is called the *product*. The symbol for multiplication is the $\times$ (multiplication or times) sign.

An important thing to know is that multiplication is a shortcut for addition:

$$
\begin{array}{rl}
4 & \text{the number of days you work at the spa} \\
\times 7 & \text{the number of hours you work each day} \\
\hline
=28 & \text{the number of hours you work each week}
\end{array}
$$

To figure out the number of hours worked at the spa in one week, you could have added the following:

$$7 + 7 + 7 + 7 = 28$$

Although adding the numbers did yield the same results, it is quicker and more efficient to multiply.

WORD CLUE

There are several words that let us know that multiplication is the correct operation for solving a problem, and they are *per*, *total*, *factors*, *twice*, *times*, and *product*.

Read the questions below and determine how to solve them before reading the answer—are your conclusions correct?

1. Maylie purchased 6 bottles of nail polish for $5 each. What is the total **cost** of the 6 bottles of polish at $5 each?

2. Ally purchased 6 boxes of foundation for $24 per box. How much did Ally pay for all the boxes of foundation?

Division

Division is the *reducing* of one or more sets of numbers. The number that is being divided is called the **dividend**, and the number that is doing the dividing is called the **divisor**. The answer that the dividend and divisor create is called the **quotient**.

An example of this concept is $28 \div 4 = 7$; the *28* is called the *dividend*, the *4* is called the *divisor*, and the *7* is called the *quotient*. The symbol for division is the $\div$ (division) sign. Division is the reverse of multiplication and a shortcut for subtraction:

28	the total number of hours you can work at the spa
$\div 4$	the total number of days you can work at the spa
$= 7$	the number of hours you need to work each of the 4 days you are at the spa

Any time a problem asks for the cost per unit, or uses words like *each*, *per*, or *quotient*, we have to divide or subtract.

Read the questions below and determine how to solve them before reading the answer—are your conclusions correct?

1. Lisa paid $100 for 5 bulbs for her laser hair-removal machine. What is the quotient of the $100 cost and the 5 bulbs?

2. One day Allen is offered a promotional deal from his supplier. If he is willing to buy 4 cases of shampoo, the supplier will sell all 4 cases for $112 instead of the regular price of $35 per case. If Allen agrees to buy all 4 cases, how much will he pay for each case? What will his per case savings be?

MATHEMATICAL PROPERTIES

Now that we have examined the operations used in mathematics, let's take a look at the properties, or rules, by which all math works. There are six important properties of which to be aware: the law of opposite numbers and the associative, commutative, distributive, identity, and inverse properties.

Remember, these properties provide guidance and direction when we are unclear as to what should be done next. This normally occurs when we are dealing with unknowns or variables that are represented by letters like "x" and "y."

Opposite Numbers and Reciprocals

Sometimes, situations come up that complicate the everyday business of working in the salon or spa, and the following mathematical properties can help you reach the correct conclusion.

The opposite of a positive number is a negative number, and, of course, the opposite of a negative number is a positive number. Positive and negative numbers are the opposite of each other because they are on the opposite side of zero on a number line.

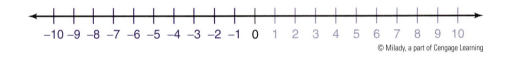

© Milady, a part of Cengage Learning

How will positive and negative numbers affect you in the salon setting? Let's say that you arrive at work one morning without any cash in your wallet. Some of your coworkers decide to order breakfast from the local deli and because you have no cash, your friend offers to lend you $5 for the breakfast special. You accept. At this point, you are at a negative cash flow for the day, –$5, because you have spent money you do not have and you need to repay your friend.

As the day comes to a close, you cash out and realize that your profits for the day are $100; however, you need to repay your friend the $5 you borrowed for breakfast:

$100	total service profits
+ –$5	amount you owe to your friend
= $95	total take-home after repaying your debt

The reciprocal (opposite) of a number is the inverted form of the number where the top part of the number and bottom part of the number change places when written in fraction form. If the number is not a fraction but a whole number, just draw a line under the number and place a 1 underneath the line to create a fraction. All whole numbers can be written in fraction form. Here's an example: The reciprocal of 5 is $\frac{1}{5}$. To achieve this we placed a 1 under the 5, like this: $\frac{5}{1}$. Now we are ready to produce the reciprocal of 5. We have not changed the value of 5 by doing this. If we were to divide 5 by 1, it would give us the number 5. All fractions are division problems waiting to happen.

This is a very important concept about fractions that we revisit a little later in this text.

1-5 LET ME TRY **Read the questions below and determine how to solve them before reading the answer—are your conclusions correct?**

1. What is the opposite of 8?

2. What is the **o**pposite of –5?

3. What is the reciprocal of $\frac{7}{1}$?

4. What is the reciprocal of $\frac{8}{12}$?

The Associative Property

The **associative property** is a property that is used with addition or multiplication, but not both at the same time. The property states that the grouping of the numbers in an equation in different arrangements does not affect the answer. In the example below, notice that the numbers in the first and second equation are all in the same place, they have not moved—only the parentheses have moved.

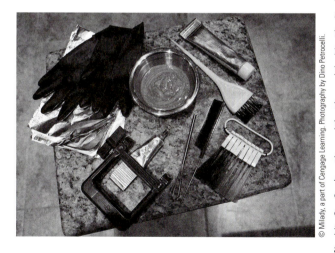

© Milady, a part of Cengage Learning. Photography by Dino Petrocelli.

When numbers are in parentheses, it indicates that the operation in the parentheses should be completed first.

In the salon, you decide upon associative properties every day—does that surprise you? Here is how: A client comes in for a haircut and color service; you can decide to cut her hair first and then color it, or to color it first and then cut it. Either way the outcome is the same: when she leaves she will have had both a haircut and a color service!

Here is what the associative property looks like in a math equation:

1st equation: $3 + (4 + 5) = 12$
2nd equation: $(3 + 4) + 5 = 12$

1–6 **LET ME TRY**

Read the questions below and determine how to solve them before reading the answer—are your conclusions correct?

1. If Jane does inventory on Tuesday, and that same day she orders 7 tubes of haircolor in one phone call and then calls back to order 3 bottles of acetone and 4 jars of polymer powder, how many items did Jane order for her spa?

2. **A.** Marty is seeing 5 clients today, and each of them is having a haircut that costs $25 and a color service that costs $45. How much will Marty's services total?

   B. If Marty can successfully upsell 2 of his clients and recommends that they purchase a duo of color-enhancing shampoo and conditioner for $25, how much will his sales total?

The Commutative Property

The **commutative property** is another property that is used with addition or multiplication, but not both at the same time. The commutative property states that moving the numbers around, or changing the order of the numbers, does not affect the answer. You can see in the example below that whether the numbers are added in the order of the first or second equation, the answer is always the same.

Again, you do this in the salon every day—think about the last time you formulated haircolor. You grabbed the bowl and a brush, a tube of color, and a bottle of developer. Does it make any difference to the color formula, and ultimately, the color service, if you pour the developer or squeeze the color into the bowl first? Of course not—the outcome is the same!

1st equation: $3 + 4 + 5 = 12$
2nd equation: $5 + 4 + 3 = 12$

1–7 **LET ME TRY**

Read the questions below and determine how to solve them before reading the answer—are your conclusions correct?

1. **A.** Barry goes to the supply store and picks up a shampoo cape ($12.99), a dozen styling combs ($6.99), and a bottle of haircolor ($3.25). He goes to check-out and the clerk rings them up. What is his total?

B. If Barry had purchased the very same items as above but the check-out clerk had rung up the bottle of haircolor first, then the dozen styling combs, and finally the shampoo cape, how much would Barry's total have been?

The Distributive Property

The **distributive property** is a property that is used with multiplication, addition, and subtraction. Multiplication and at least one of the other operations must be present. The distributive property states that we multiply the number on the outside of the parentheses by everything that is on the inside of the parentheses, completing the operation in the parentheses first; this is called the *order of operations*.

Although we are not ready to talk about the rule of the order of operation yet, here is a sneak peak. The rule of the **order of operations** declares that when there are different operations in a problem they must be completed in a specific order. The order is parentheses, exponents, multiplication, division, addition, and subtraction (PEMDAS). We use the acronym PEMDAS, which is formed by the first letter in each word, to remember the order. We discuss this in greater depth later in the book.

In order to complete this equation $3 \times (4 + 5)$, you would complete the equation inside the parentheses first, $4 + 5 = 9$, and then multiply that number by 3: $3 \times 9 = 27$.

How do you use the distributive property in your work every day? Here is how— you take a look at your schedule and see that you have 4 clients, each coming in for a manicure and pedicure. To determine your service total for the day, you add together the price of the manicure [$25] and the price of the pedicure [$35] and then multiply that number by the number of clients you will service (4). It looks like this:

4 (number of clients) $\times$ (manicure [$25] + pedicure [$35])

OR

$4 \times (\$25 + \$35) = \$240$

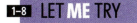 **1-8 LET ME TRY**

Read the questions below and determine how to solve them before reading the answer—are your conclusions correct?

1. **A.** On Monday morning Gina has 2 UV gel nail services scheduled. She charges $35 for each. On Monday afternoon she has 3 manicures and a pedicure scheduled, for which she charges $25 for the manicures and $30 for the pedicure. How much will her services total on Monday?

B. On Tuesday morning, Gina is scheduled to perform 3 manicures at $25 each and a pedicure at $30. In the afternoon she is scheduled to perform 2 polymer powder and monomer liquid nail enhancement services for $35 each. How much will her service total be on Tuesday? Did Gina make more money on Monday or Tuesday?

2. A. The Derma Brilliance Spa is running a special. If a client brings in the postcard that was mailed to them, they get $10 off any service that costs $50 or more. The estheticians are excited because the mailer has generated lots of interest and their schedules are full. Monica's schedule indicates that she has 4 clients that day, and each is booked for a **one** hour facial, priced at $80. How much will Monica's service total be?

B. If Monica also recommends a paraffin wax treatment to her clients, which costs an additional $22, and two of her clients agree to have it, how much **will** Monica's total **be** now?

Identity Property

The **identity property** is a property that is used with addition or multiplication. The identity property states that when zero is added to a number or when a number is multiplied by one, it does not change the original number. Zero is the identity number for addition, and one is the identity number for multiplication:

addition: $8 + 0 = 8$
multiplication: $8 \times 1 = 8$

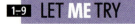 **1-9 LET ME TRY**

Read the questions below and determine how to solve them before reading the answer—are your conclusions correct?

1. Patty has advertised her new salon in the local newspaper for the first time. In the ad it states that if the client mentions reading about the salon in the newspaper, **she** will receive a 25 percent savings on **her** services that day. Patty has seen 5 clients since the ad has run, but none have mentioned the ad. How many clients has she seen?

2. Tim has decided that he needs to hire a full-time receptionist instead of relying on stylists to answer the phone, make appointments, and help clients. He has enough money to hire 1 receptionist for the 52 weeks of the upcoming year. How many weeks will his salon have a receptionist?

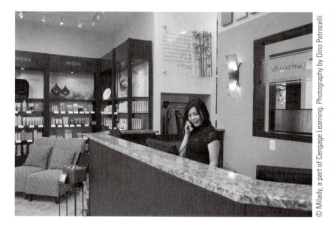

© Milady, a part of Cengage Learning. Photography by Dino Petrocelli.

Inverse Property

The **inverse property** is a property that is used with addition or multiplication. The inverse property of addition states that any time you add a number to its opposite the answer is zero. The inverse property of multiplication states that any time you multiply a number by its reciprocal (opposite) the answer is 1.

Remember that zero and one, respectively, are the identity numbers for addition and multiplication.

addition: $8 + (-8) = 0$

multiplication: $8 \times \frac{1}{8} = 1$

1–10 LET ME TRY

Read the questions below and determine how to solve them before reading the answer—are your conclusions correct?

1. Anton ordered 24 tubes of spiking glue at the beginning of the week, and by the end of the week he realizes that he has sold 12 tubes of spiking glue and that 3 tubes were returned to the salon for a refund because they were leaking and gooey. How many tubes of spiking glue does Anton have on hand to sell?

REVIEW QUESTIONS

Note: The answer key to chapter review questions is found at the back of the book.

1. Define mathematics and name the four mathematical operations used in problem-solving.

2. In the equation $7 + 2 = 9$, which number(s) represents the addends and which number(s) represents the sum?

3. List the key words within a problem that indicate addition is the proper operation to use to solve it.

4. In the equation $9 - 2 = 7$, which number(s) represents the minuend, which number(s) represents the subtrahend, and which number(s) represents the difference?

5. List the key words within a problem that indicate subtraction is the proper operation to use to solve it.

6. In the equation $3 \times 2 = 6$, which number(s) represents the factors and which number(s) represents the product?

7. List the key words within a problem that indicate multiplication is the proper operation to use to solve it.

8. In the equation $6 \div 2 = 3$, which number(s) represents the dividend, which number(s) represents the divisor, and which number(s) represent the quotient?

9. List the key words within a problem that indicate division is the proper operation to use to solve it.

10. Name at least three ways beauty and wellness professionals can use the four mathematical operations in their every day work.

11. What is an opposite number? Give an example of how it can be useful.

12. Define and explain the associative property.

13. Define and explain the commutative property.

14. Define and explain the distributive property.

15. Define and explain the identity property.

16. Define and explain the inverse property.

Appointment Planning and Scheduling Clients

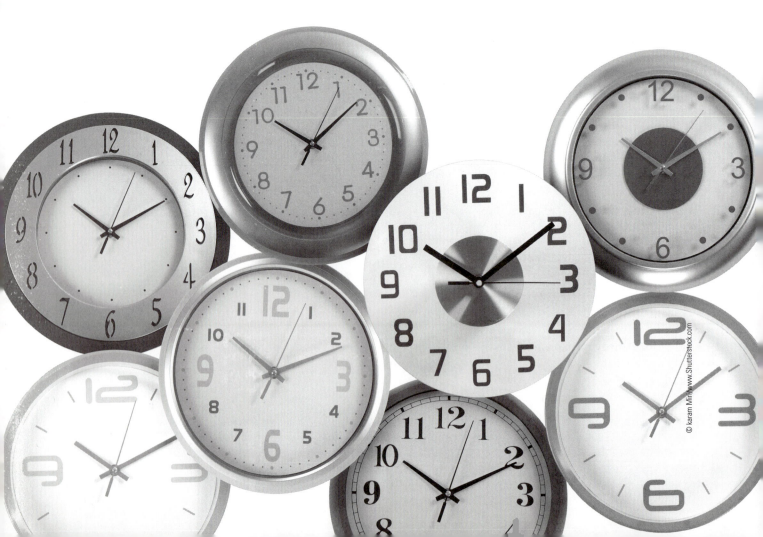

- The Mathematics of Appointment Planning
- Making Your Appointment Calendar Work for You

LEARNING OBJECTIVES

After completing this chapter, you will be able to:

1. Know and understand the importance of efficiently scheduling clients and appointments.

2. Name and identify how integers are used in the appointment scheduling process.

3. Identify and explain how fractions are used in the appointment scheduling process.

4. Make determinations about your workday and work hours that will lead to effective scheduling.

5. Know and use the rules of adding integers to plan your schedule.

6. Know and use the rules of subtracting integers to plan your schedule.

7. Know and use the rules of multiplying integers to plan your schedule.

8. Know and use the rules of dividing integers to plan your schedule.

KEY TERMS

- fractions
- integers
- negative numbers
- point of origin
- positive numbers
- sign
- signed number

NE OF THE MOST IMPORTANT ACTIVITIES ACCOMPLISHED IN THE SALON OR spa each day is…appointment planning or scheduling! Scheduling is the lifeblood of the salon and spa business—it is the schedule through which your revenue stream comes into and goes out of the business. So scheduling smartly is an imperative goal. Whether you use an automated system for your scheduling, an online scheduling program, or the tried-and-true paper appointment book, making the best, wisest use of your time while at work is one good way to ensure that your business remains financially secure.

THE MATHEMATICS OF APPOINTMENT PLANNING

As we have already discussed, making and keeping a schedule of appointments is very important. Equally as important is knowing how much time you have and can spend with each client and the total time it takes to complete each service—these are vital first steps to successful scheduling. Clients want to receive good, competent services, but they also want their time to be respected by their practitioner, and they deserve to be treated that way.

In order to create your schedule, you need to determine the total hours that are available in a day and then subtract the time that you need to spend with each customer, plus a few extra minutes for consultation and preparation time. Doing all that by subtraction can be time-consuming, so we are going to explore using integers to change subtraction into addition and move things around so that you get the same answer in a lot less time.

Integers

Integers are positive or negative whole numbers like 1, 2, and 3, which are positive numbers, and −1, −2, and −3, which are negative numbers.

Positive numbers reside on the right side of zero on a number line. Positive numbers are the opposite of negative numbers. Words that clue us in to know that a number is positive are *gained, up, increased, right, plus, available,* and *good.*

Negative numbers reside on the left side of zero on a number line. Negative numbers are the opposite of positive numbers. Words that clue us in to know that a number is negative are *lost, down, decreased, left, subtract, used,* and *bad.*

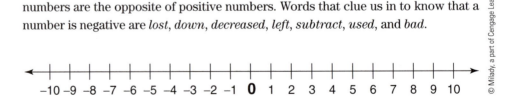

Because the starting point for all measurement begins with zero, zero is called the **point of origin.** The point of origin is where a measurement begins. Zero is the point of origin for all numbers. The farther a number is away from zero on the right

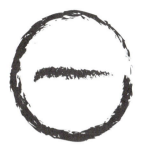
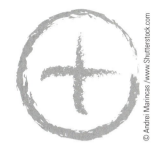

side of a number line, the *larger* the number. The farther a number is away from zero on the left side of a number line, the *smaller* the number. All positive numbers are to the right of zero and all negative numbers are to the left of zero.

When there is a symbol in front of a number that allows us to know whether the number is negative or positive, it is called a **sign**. The positive signs are often invisible, whereas negative signs are always visible.

Example 1: $3 + 6 = 9$ (In this equation, because no signs are present, we can assume that these are all positive numbers.)

Example 2: $3 + -6 = -3$ (In this equation, we have to add a negative number to a positive number; in this case, the answer to the equation is negative.)

When a number is positive, indicated by a $+$ sign, or negative, indicated by a $-$ sign, it is called a **signed number**, thus indicating which side of the number line it resides on. Signed numbers can be fractions and decimals as well as whole numbers.

Zero is an integer, but it is not a signed number because it is neither positive nor negative.

DID YOU KNOW? Negative numbers are synonymous with the operation of subtraction, and positive numbers are synonymous with the operation of addition.

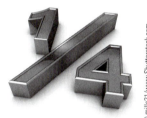

Fractions

Because not every procedure or service you perform takes exactly 1 hour to complete, we need to take a look at the mathematical concept of fractions.

Fractions count a portion or piece of something; a fraction is a ratio that compares two numbers by division, or we could say that every fraction is a division problem waiting to happen. There is a top and a bottom number for every fraction, written, for example, as $\frac{1}{2}$. Although we delve into fractions more deeply in the next chapter, we need to use them in schedule planning in a very specific way.

You want to make the best use of your time in a day, and so you need to schedule your appointments based on the actual time it may take to perform a service. Imagine if you could only schedule services every hour. How many services do you perform that only take you 45 minutes to accomplish? If you could only schedule services every hour, you would be wasting the remaining 15 minutes every time you performed a 45-minute service. That could add up to a lot of unnecessary wasted time in your schedule.

So, in the case of an hour, we can say that it contains 4 parts—every 15 minutes of an hour is 1 part, so one 15-minute segment of an hour would be expressed as $\frac{1}{4}$.

Planning the Schedule

So, now you are ready to work on your appointment calendar for the week. There are a few variables you have to determine before you can start making those appointments.

First, how many days per week will you be working? Next, how many hours per day will you work? Third, how long does it take for you to complete basic services, on average? Use the worksheet below to answer these questions.

Use the table below to fill in answers that reflect your work schedule and the services you perform.

Q: How many days per week will I be working?	A:
Q: How many hours per day will I be working?	A:
Q: How long does it take me to complete a client consultation, shampoo, haircut, and styling, on average?	A:
Q: How long does it take me to complete a client consultation, one-process haircoloring, haircut, and styling, on average?	A:
Q: How long does it take me to complete a client consultation, foiling, trim, and styling, on average?	A:
Q: How long does it take me to complete a client consultation, permanent wave, trim, and styling, on average?	A:
Q: How long does it take me to complete a client consultation, chemical relaxing service, trim, and styling, on average?	A:
Q: How long does it take me to complete a client consultation, wet set, and comb-out, on average?	A:

MAKING YOUR APPOINTMENT CALENDAR WORK FOR YOU

Knowing that excellent planning and scheduling are important to both you and your clients, you should take some time to create an appointment calendar that

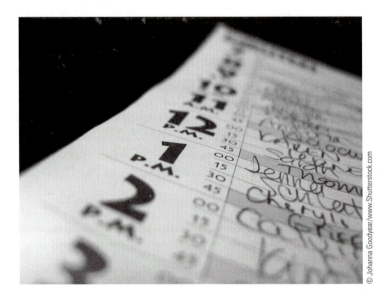

works well for you. Be sure to schedule a lunch break during the day so that you can eat and rest a bit, and be sure to have other scheduled times in your calendar to attend to your personal grooming needs and to refresh your own professional look/image.

Although you may be tempted to "fit in" a good, loyal, or long-time client or to cut some corners, run late, or run-over while doing services to accommodate additional client requests, be sure not to do this too often because it disrupts your well-planned scheduling process as well as indicates to clients that their schedule times and appointments aren't "real" anyway.

There are a several ways to accommodate client requests for extra services without infringing on your carefully planned appointment calendar. Here are a couple of solutions to consider:

- If a client requests an additional or unexpected service, check to see whether it can be done immediately. If it can, then of course you should do it.
- If the additional service cannot be done immediately, suggest she return at a time when it can be comfortably fit into the schedule.
- If you cannot perform the service, determine whether a colleague can perform the service for you.
- Finally, suggest that she make an appointment exclusively for that service and schedule it as soon as possible.

Scheduling Appointments

Now it is time for you to begin scheduling your day. You are going to be working with signed numbers—positive and negative—and remember: If a number does not have a sign, it is a positive number.

Using the following table, and knowing that positive numbers are considered available hours and negative numbers are considered used hours, answer the questions in the following "Show Me How".

Q: How many days per week will I be working?	A: 5 days—Tuesday through Saturday
Q: How many hours per day will I be working?	A: 8 hours (from 8 a.m. to 5 p.m.), including a 1-hour lunch break from 12 p.m. to 1 p.m.
Q: How long does it take me to complete a client consultation, shampoo, haircut, and styling, on average?	A: 1 hour
Q: How long does it take me to complete a client consultation, one-process haircoloring, haircut and styling, on average?	A: 2 hours
Q: How long does it take me to complete a client consultation, foiling, trim, and styling on average?	A: $2\frac{1}{2}$ hours
Q: How long does it take me to complete a client consultation, permanent wave, trim, and styling on average?	A: 3 hours
Q: How long does it take me to complete a client consultation, chemical relaxing service, trim, and styling on average?	A: 3 hours
Q: How long does it take me to complete a client consultation, wet set, and comb-out on average?	A: $1\frac{1}{2}$ hours
Q: How long does it take me to complete a client consultation, blowdry, and thermal styling on average?	A: $1\frac{1}{2}$ hours
Q: How long does it take me to complete a client consultation and facial, on average?	A: 1 hour
Q: How long does it take me to complete a client consultation and manicure, on average?	A: 45 minutes

QUESTION 1: You have 8 hours available to schedule appointments on Tuesday. Your appointment book shows that you have 3 haircuts scheduled. How much time do you have left to schedule other appointments after you have completed the 3 haircut appointments?

ANSWER: You have 8 available hours each day, but 3 of those hours will be lost due to appointments. The equation would look like this:

8	hours in a workday
$+ -3$	scheduled appointments
$= 5$	hours still available for taking appointments

QUESTION 2: **A.** It is Friday and you have a pretty full day of appointments. You have a perm and a one-process haircoloring already scheduled. A client calls and wants to book a haircut and a manicure. Your haircolor client asks whether she can add a facial to her service that day. Are you able to accommodate all of these requests?

ANSWER: You must now figure out how much available time there is and subtract all of the appointment times to see how your schedule can accommodate the client's requests. We have to do it in 2 steps.

STEP 1:

8	hours in the workday
$+ -3$	time it takes to complete a perm service
$= 5$	hours left in the day

5	hours left in the day
$+ -2$	time it takes to complete a one-process haircolor service
$= 3$	hours left in the day to schedule services

STEP 2: Now you take the remaining hours left in your schedule and see which of the new services you can add.

3	remaining hours in the day to schedule services
$+ -1$	time it takes to perform a facial for your haircolor client
$= 2$	hours left in the day to schedule services

2	hours left in the day to schedule services
$+ -1\frac{3}{4}$	time it takes to perform a haircut and manicure service
$= 15$	number of minutes left in your scheduled work day

B. Did any of the services have to be scheduled for another day?

ANSWER: No, they did not.

QUESTION 3: **A.** On Thursday, you have signed-up for a class at your local distributor's education center. The class begins at 9 a.m. and ends at 12 p.m. You then head to the salon and complete the workday. It takes you half an hour to get to the salon from the education center, so how much time is available for scheduling appointments?

ANSWER:

8	number of hours in a work day
$+ -3\frac{1}{2}$	number of hours unavailable to schedule clients
$= 4\frac{1}{2}$	number of hours available for scheduling clients

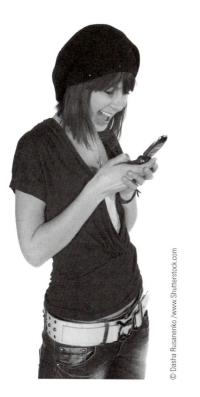

© Dasha Rusanenko /www.Shutterstock.com

B. While at the class, you receive a text from the salon's receptionist that says two clients have called in to make appointments for that day. One client wants to book a chemical relaxing service and the other wants to have a shampoo, blowdry, and thermal styling for an event she is attending that evening. The receptionist asks you whether she can schedule the clients. After completing the following calculations, what information will you text her back?

ANSWER:

12:30	the time you will arrive at the salon
$4\frac{1}{2}$	number of hours available for scheduling clients
+ −3	number of hours it will take to perform a chemical relaxing service
+ −$1\frac{1}{2}$	number of hours it will take to perform a shampoo, blowdry, and thermal styling
= 0	number of hours left to schedule appointments

The receptionist can book these two appointments for today, but any other requests have to be scheduled for another day.

QUESTION 4: As you examine your appointment book you realize that you do not have any appointments scheduled for Wednesday, and there are 3 hours on Thursday that are available for scheduling appointments also. How many total hours do you have available to schedule appointments between those two days?

ANSWER:

8	hours available on Wednesday
+ 3	hours available on Thursday
= 11	total number of hours available for scheduling

Adding or Subtracting?

When working with integers, how can you be sure when to add and when to subtract? Keep in mind that positive numbers are considered *available* hours and negative numbers (numbers with a minus sign) are considered *used* hours. In the question above, you had 8 available hours on Wednesday and 3 available hours on Thursday, so to find out how many total hours you have available for scheduling appointments we added the two numbers to get the answer: $8 + 3 = 11$.

In this question, both integers are positive with an addition sign in between them. You do not need to follow any special rules here—all you have to do is to add the numbers together.

Adding Integers

There are some rules you have to be aware of, however, when adding integers.

- **Adding Rule 1:** When adding integers, if the numbers have the same sign, add the numbers and attach the sign of the larger digit. This is called the *same sign sum*.

$8 + 3 = 11$

- **Adding Rule 2:** When adding integers that have different signs find the *difference* between (subtract) the numbers and attach the sign of the larger digit. This is called the *different sign difference*.

$$11 + -8 = 3$$

Within the question, there are words that help clue you in to which operation you need to use—addition or subtraction.

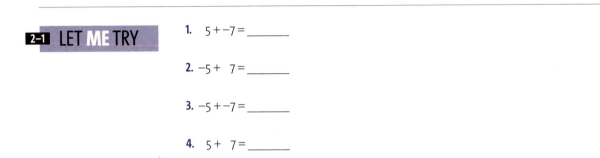

2-1 LET ME TRY

1. $5 + -7 =$ _____

2. $-5 + 7 =$ _____

3. $-5 + -7 =$ _____

4. $5 + 7 =$ _____

Subtracting Integers

Subtracting integers can get a little trickier—remember that negative numbers are considered used hours, and used hours have to be *subtracted* from available hours in order to know how much time is available for scheduling.

As with adding integers, there is a special rule to keep in mind when subtracting integers:

> **Subtracting Integers Rule:** Never subtract negative integers. Change the subtraction sign to addition, then change the sign of the number following the addition sign to its opposite, and last but not least follow the rule for adding integers with the same signs or different signs.

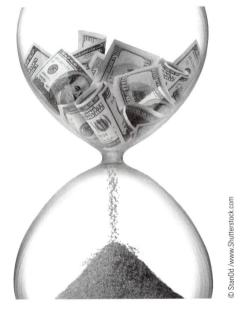

Note that it takes a change to offset a change. There are always two changes. This is an important math skill. It is revisited a little later when we discuss dealing with fractions and division. We can rewrite a problem and change its operation as long as we remember to make two changes. This is called *change, change*.

Within the question, there are words that help clue you in to which operation you need to use—addition or subtraction.

QUESTION 1:   At the beginning of the week you had 9 hours available to schedule appointments. On Tuesday, 3 of your 1-hour appointments called and canceled. If you remove the canceled appointments from your appointment book, how many hours do you have available to schedule appointments for the remainder of the week?

ANSWER: Remember that positive numbers are considered available hours, and you had 9 hours available at the beginning of the week. On Tuesday 3 hours were taken away from the hours that were already scheduled for appointments; therefore, you should subtract or take away the lost time. The equation looks like this: $9 - (-3) = 12$.

STEP 1: Change the subtraction sign to an addition sign.
$9 + (-3)$

STEP 2: Change the number following the addition sign to its opposite.
$9 + (+3)$

STEP 3: Follow the Rule for Adding Integers with the same sign.
$9 + 3 = 12$

QUESTION 2:   You are scheduled to style the hair for several people in the same wedding party on Saturday, and you also have a full book of appointments that day. Marcy, the bride's mother, calls to add herself and her other daughter Ashley (who is also in the wedding) to your list for that day—how can you say no? They both need a blowdry and styling. You know that the bridesmaids are wearing flowers in their hair, so Ashley needs a shampoo, blowdry, updo, and flowers have to be added to the completed style—you figure this will take an extra half-hour.
How much time is left for you to schedule additional clients that day?

ANSWER:
8	number of hours available on Saturday
-8	number of hours already scheduled on Saturday
$= 0$	number of hours left to schedule appointments

0 number of hours left on Saturday to schedule appointments

-1	amount of time a shampoo, blowdry, and styling for Marcy will take
$-1\frac{1}{2}$	amount of time a shampoo, blowdry, updo, and flower placement for Ashley will take
$= -2\frac{1}{2}$	amount of time that you are overbooked for Saturday

QUESTION 3:   Due to a personal emergency, you have to be out of work on Thursday, so you have 8 hours of appointments that cannot be kept. The receptionist takes a look at your schedule and sees that you have 4 one-hour slots open for the remaining days that week. She is able to reschedule all 4 of the open one-hour appointments. How many hours still need to be rescheduled?

ANSWER:
-8	number of hours that you are overbooked
$+4$	number of hour-long appointments rescheduled into the week
$= 4$	number of hours that still need to be rescheduled

QUESTION 4: You have 9 hours available to schedule appointments at the start of the week. On Wednesday, 3 one-hour appointments were canceled. How many hours for appointments do you now have to schedule for the remainder of the week?

ANSWER:

9	number of hours you originally had open for scheduling appointments
− (− 3)	number of hour-long appointments that were canceled
= 12	number of hours now available for scheduling

STEP 1: Change the subtraction sign to an addition sign.

$(9) + (-3)$

STEP 2: Change the number following the addition sign to its opposite.

$(9) + (+3)$

STEP 3: Follow the Rule for Adding Integers with different signs.

$(9) + (+3) = 12$

Multiplying or Dividing?

Although addition and subtraction are very important, there may be a time when you will have to multiply and divide when working on your appointment scheduling. One golden rule to keep in mind regarding the multiplication and division of integers is … that if the signs are *different* in the problem, the answer is *negative*, and if the signs are the *same* in the problem, the answer is *positive*.

For example, Markee's salon has just brought in a new retail line, and he and his salon colleagues took a 4-hour training class on the products. All of the staff have committed to make a quick, 5-minute presentation of the line to each client they will service on Friday—as a means of kick-starting the salon's retail sales of the product line. When Markee looks at his appointment book, he realizes that he is fully booked on Friday. How much time does Markee actually need to add to the schedule if he intends to give each client a 5-minute presentation on the product line?

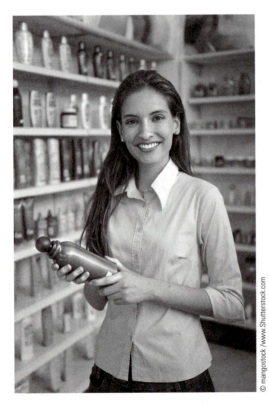

© mangostock /www.Shutterstock.com

Multiplying Integers

The easiest way to get the answer to Markee's scheduling dilemma is to multiply the amount of time he will discuss the product line by the number of clients he will see on Friday. So, the equation would look like this:

−5	number of additional minutes Markee will add to each appointment to discuss the retail line with each client
× 8	the number of clients Markee has booked for Friday
= −40	the number of minutes that Markee is overbooked on Friday

Here is the rationale for how to complete this equation:

STEP 1: Check to see whether the signs in the problem are the same or different.

−5 and 8 have different signs

STEP 2: Multiply the numbers together.

$5 \times 8 = 40$

STEP 3: Since the signs are *different* the answer is *negative*.

$-5 \times 8 = -40$

Since multiplication is a shortcut for addition, we can use addition to prove that we solved this problem correctly. The equation would look like this:

$-5 + -5 + -5 + -5 + -5 + -5 + -5 + -5 = -40$

In this example, since the signs are the same, we add the numbers and attach the sign that is in the problem after we have completed the addition of the numbers.

SHOW ME HOW

QUESTION 1: Markee decides not to devote the same 5 minutes of explanation to each of his clients on Saturday, but Sara, the receptionist, mistakenly schedules 5 extra minutes for each of the 8 clients that were scheduled. What does Sara need to do to correct the mistake, and how would the appointment book change?

ANSWER: Markee did not use 5 additional minutes for each of the 8 clients that came in on Saturday. So the additional time had to be removed or taken away for each of the 8 clients.

$(-5) \times (-8) = 40$

STEP 1: Check to see if the signs in the problem are the same or different.

−5 and −8 have the same signs

STEP 2: Multiply the numbers together.

$-5 \times -8 = 40$

STEP 3: Since the signs are the same the answer is positive.

$(-5) \times (-8) = 40$

We could prove that we solved this problem correctly through the use of subtraction, because subtraction is the reverse of addition.

STEP 1: $- (-5) - (-5) - (-5) - (-5) - (-5) - (-5) - (-5) - (-5) = 40$

STEP 2: $+ (+5) + (+5) + (+5) + (+5) + (+5) + (+5) + (+5) + (+5) = 40$

Remember, we do not subtract negative numbers, so we change the subtraction operation to addition, and we change the sign of each number following each subtraction sign to its opposite.

QUESTION 2: Angel has 6 appointments scheduled this week. Each appointment will take 2 hours including preparation time. How much total time does Angel need to complete all of the scheduled appointments for this week?

ANSWER:

2	number of hours spent per appointment
× 6	number of clients to be serviced
= 12	number of hours needed to complete all of the appointments

---

Dividing Integers

Sometimes you need to find the difference between certain numbers or you need to know how much time may be left in your schedule for making appointments; in that case, division can make all of the difference. Remember that division is a quicker way of subtracting.

SHOW ME HOW

QUESTION 1: Mary used 8 hours to complete 4 appointments. How much time, on average, did Mary use for each appointment?

ANSWER:
$$\begin{array}{ll} 8 & \text{total number of hours used to perform services} \\ \div\,4 & \text{number of appointments performed} \\ \hline = 2 & \text{number of hours each of the 4 clients received} \end{array}$$

QUESTION 2: Mary has 10 hours of available appointment time remaining in the week. If there are 5 clients that wish to schedule appointments, how much time can Mary give to each client, on average?

ANSWER:
$$\begin{array}{ll} 10 & \text{number of available hours} \\ \div\,5 & \text{number of clients wishing to make an appointment} \\ \hline = 2 & \text{average amount of time Mary can spend with each client} \end{array}$$

Note: Both integers are positive with a division sign in-between them. Because the signs are the same, all that is required is to simply divide the numbers.

DID YOU KNOW?

Multiplication and division have the same rule regarding signed numbers. If the signs are *different* in the problem, the answer is *negative*. If the signs are the *same* in the problem, the answer is *positive*.

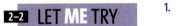 **LET ME TRY**

1. $7 \times (-5) =$ _____

2. $(-7) \times (-5) =$ _____

3. $35 \div (-7) =$ _____

4. $(-35) \div (-7) =$ _____

1. Why is it important to a salon or spa professional to efficiently schedule clients and appointments?

2. What are integers, and how are they used in the appointment scheduling process?

3. What are fractions, and how are they used in the appointment scheduling process?

4. What are the most important rules for adding integers? How can they help you in appointment planning?

5. What are the most important rules for subtracting integers? How can they help you in appointment planning?

6. What are the most important rules for multiplying integers? How can they help you in appointment planning?

7. What are the most important rules for dividing integers? How can they help you in appointment planning?

Inventory Control and Management

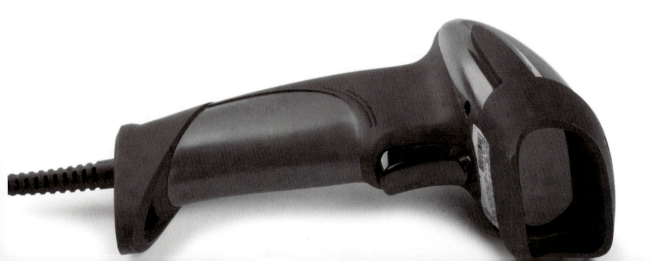

- Fractions
- Adding and Subtracting Fractions
- Multiplying and Dividing Fractions

LEARNING OBJECTIVES

After completing this chapter, you will be able to:

1. Identify and define fractions.

2. Simplify fractions to create useable numbers for inventory control.

3. Know what equivalent fractions are and use them in inventory management.

4. Add and subtract fractions with like denominators.

5. Add and subtract fractions with unlike denominators.

6. Multiply and divide fractions using the greatest common factor method.

7. Multiply fractions using the cross-canceling method.

8. Divide fractions without using the cross-canceling method.

9. Divide fractions using the cross-canceling method.

KEY TERMS

- composite number
- cross-canceling
- denominator
- equivalent fraction
- factor
- fraction
- greatest common factor (GCF)

- greatest common factor method
- least common denominator or multiple (LCM)
- like denominator fractions
- numerator
- prime factorization

- prime fraction
- prime number
- reciprocal
- simplified fraction
- unlike denominator fractions

N AREA OF GREAT SIGNIFICANCE FOR A SALON OR SPA IS ITS INVENTORY management. Having the correct amount of inventory and knowing when and how much to order is not only important for the salon's ability to service clients, but it also can have a great impact on cash flow. Order too much and you can watch inventory sit on the shelf generating no cash flow—tying up assets that could be used for other things; order too little and you may find yourself in a position to be short on vital products and unable to service and sell to clients.

Once you learn about fractions and how to work with them, counting your current inventory and planning for purchasing inventory will be more efficient and less time-consuming for everyone in the salon or spa.

FRACTIONS

The best way to manage inventory is to know what inventory you have on hand. This may be easier said than done, because, well, inventory can get messy. Take a moment to look around your school, salon, or spa—what do you see? Most likely, you will find partially used bottles, cans, and tubes of supplies—right?

Look at the new shipment of color that just came in to the salon—are the tubes packed in six-packs? Do you buy shampoo by the gallon or by the case? Do you see

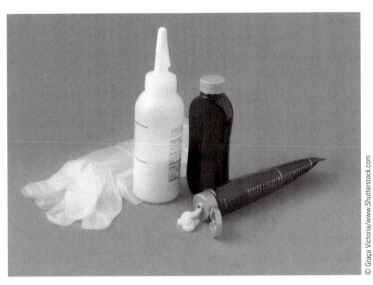

a plethora of various types of styling aids strewn around the cutting floor, all used to some degree? How, then, can an accurate inventory be taken in a circumstance such as this?

In the previous chapters, we have concentrated on whole numbers and completing mathematical operations with whole numbers—but now we are going to explore counting a portion or piece of something; these are called fractions. A **fraction** is a ratio (the relationship in quantity, amount, or size between two or more things) that compares two numbers by dividing one into the other. A fraction is a division problem waiting to happen. There is a top and a bottom number for every fraction.

The top number of a fraction is called the **numerator**. The numerator represents the amount that is chosen, taken, used, received, or given.

The bottom number of a fraction is called the **denominator**. The denominator represents the total amount of pieces or parts.

So, for example, let's say that you purchased and have used 12 ounces (336 grams) of a 16-ounce (448-gram) container of powdered bleach. What fraction represents the amount of bleach used? Keep in mind that 12 ounces (224 grams) was the amount used, so it is the numerator, or top number, and 16 ounces (448 grams) represents the total amount of the can of bleach, so it is the denominator. The fraction that represents this example is $\frac{12}{16}$.

Let's take a look at some word problems and convert them into numerical problems using fractions. Follow these steps to determine the correct fraction:

STEP 1: Identify the numerator.

STEP 2: Identify the denominator.

STEP 3: Write the fraction by putting the numerator over the denominator.

SHOW ME HOW

QUESTION 1: Bob received 2 awards out of the 7 awards that were given at the U.S. Hair Styling Championships. What fraction represents the amount of awards that Bob received?

ANSWER:

2   the number of awards Bob received (numerator)

7   the total number of awards given (denominator)

$= \dfrac{2}{7}$ the fraction that represents how many awards Bob won of the total awards given

QUESTION 2: Of the 8 clients John saw on Monday, 3 received a haircut. What fraction represents the total number of haircuts given by John on Monday?

ANSWER:

3   the number of clients who received haircuts (numerator)

8   the total number of clients John saw on Monday (denominator)

$= \dfrac{3}{8}$ the fraction that represents how many of John's clients on Monday received haircuts

QUESTION 3: On her break, Brenda bought a candy bar and divided it into 9 pieces. She gave Amanda 4 pieces of the candy bar and kept the rest for herself. What fraction represents the amount of candy that Brenda kept for herself?

ANSWER:

5   the number of pieces of the candy bar that Brenda kept for herself (numerator)

9   the total number of pieces the candy bar was broken into (denominator)

$= \dfrac{5}{9}$ the fraction that represents how much of the candy bar Brenda kept for herself

QUESTION 4: Juan notices that 8 ounces (236.56 milliliters) of shampoo were left in a 32-ounce (946.24-milliliter) bottle. What fraction represents the amount of shampoo that was left in the bottle?

ANSWER:

8   the number of ounces of shampoo left in the bottle (numerator)

32   the total amount of shampoo that was available in the bottle of shampoo (denominator)

$= \dfrac{8}{32}$ the fraction that represents how much shampoo is left in the bottle

---

As we continue to explore fractions and how to work with them, there are a few more key terms and concepts for you to be aware of.

A **factor** is a number that can divide into another number and create an answer that is a whole number without a remainder. For example, 7 is a *factor* of 21 because if you divide 21 by 7 the answer will be the whole number 3.

A factor can also be two numbers that you multiply together to come up with a total. The numbers 7 and 3 are the *factors* of 21 because if you multiply 7 and 3 together they will equal 21.

A **prime number** is a number that is divisible only by 1 and itself. An example of a prime number is the number 7 because there are only two factors that can be divided into 7, 1 and 7.

Prime numbers are odd numbers except for the number 2, which is the only even number that is a prime number. Examples of prime numbers are 2, 3, 5, 7, 11, 13, 17, 19, 23, 29, 31, 37, and so on.

If a fraction has a prime number for a numerator and a prime number for a denominator, it cannot be simplified or reduced.

A **composite number** is a number that is divisible by more than 1 and itself, like the number 9. Nine can be divided by 1, 3, or 9 because $1 \times 9 = 9$ and $3 \times 3 = 9$. A composite number can be odd or even. In order for a fraction to be simplified or reduced, the denominator, the numerator, or both must be a composite number. More examples of composite numbers are 4, 6, 8, 9, 10, 12, 15, 16, 18, 20, 21, and so forth.

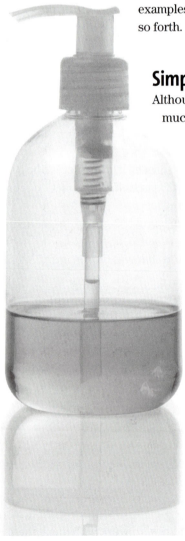

Simplifying Fractions

Although Juan, in the example earlier in this chapter, now knows how much shampoo is left in the bottle $\left(\frac{8}{32}\right)$ trying to count inventory using a fraction like $\frac{8}{32}$ is pretty difficult to manage, so it would be wise to simplify the fraction by reducing large numbers to make them smaller and easier to manage. Simplifying fractions also allows us to add and subtract fractions.

So, a **simplified fraction** is obtained when we *divide* the numerator and the denominator of a fraction by the same number.

An **equivalent fraction** is when two fractions look different but have the same value and are obtained when we either multiply or divide the numerator and the denominator of a fraction by the same number. Fractions, like money, can look different but have the same value. For example, four $5 bills are equal to one $20 bill, and one $20 bill is equal to two $10 bills, but they look very different.

A **prime fraction** is obtained when a fraction cannot be simplified. One example of this is the fraction $\frac{1}{2}$.

The **greatest common factor (GCF)** is the *largest* number that we can divide two or more numbers by. The greatest common factor's primary focal point is division.

The **least common denominator or multiple (LCM)** is the *smallest* number that two numbers share in common if we are multiplying or counting by both numbers. The least common multiple's primary focal point is multiplication.

© Atiketta Sangasaeng/www.Shutterstock.com

QUESTION 1: Annie used 12 ounces (336 grams) of a 16-ounce (448-gram) container of powdered bleach. How much powdered bleach did Annie use?

ANSWER: **STEP 1:** Determine the fraction that represents how much bleach was used.

$\quad$ 12 $\quad$ the numerator

$\quad$ 16 $\quad$ the denominator

$\quad = \dfrac{12}{16} \quad$ the fraction

STEP 2: To make this number really useable and understandable, we must find the greatest common factor, or the largest number we can divide both the numerator and the denominator by. To determine this, we must list all the factors of 12 and 16. This can be done through the use of division or multiplication. We could say what two numbers multiplied together equal 12, or we could ask what number can 12 be divided by?

$\quad 3 \times 4 = 12$

$\quad 12 \div 3 = 4$

thus, 3 and 4 are factors of 12

STEP 3: Find the largest factor of the numerator and the denominator.

$\quad$ 1, 2, 3, 4, 6, and 12 $\quad$ factors of the numerator 12

$\quad$ 1, 2, 4, 8, and 16 $\quad$ factors of the denominator 12

STEP 4: Determine the greatest common factor (GCF).

$\quad$ 4 $\quad$ the greatest common factor of 12 and 16

STEP 5: Divide the numerator and the denominator by the greatest common factor.

$\quad \dfrac{12}{16} \div 4$

$\quad$ or

$\quad \dfrac{12 \div 4}{16 \div 4} = \dfrac{3}{4}$

When Annie used 12 ounces (336 grams) of a 16-ounce (448-gram) container of powdered bleach, she actually used $\frac{3}{4}$ of the container. The fraction $\frac{3}{4}$ is a much easier fraction to work with than $\frac{12}{16}$ is.

QUESTION 2: Mattie had 8ounces (236.56 milliliters) of a 16-ounce (473.12-milliliter) bottle of shampoo left after she completed all her appointments for the day. How much shampoo does Mattie have left?

ANSWER: **STEP 1:** Write the fraction.

$\quad$ 8 $\quad$ number of ounces of shampoo left in the bottle (numerator)

$\quad$ 16 $\quad$ total number of ounces of shampoo available in the bottle (denominator)

$\quad \dfrac{8}{16} \quad$ fraction representing how much shampoo is left at the end of the day

STEP 2: Identify the factors (divisors) of the numerator and the denominator.

$\quad$ 1, 2, 4, and 8 $\quad$ the factors of 8

$\quad$ 1, 2, 4, 8, and 16 $\quad$ the factors of 16

STEP 3: Determine the greatest common factor of the numerator and the denominator.

8   the greatest common factor of 8 and 16

STEP 4: Divide the numerator and the denominator by the greatest common factor.

$$\frac{8 \div 8}{16 \div 8} = \frac{1}{2}$$

When Mattie had 8 ounces (236.56 milliliters) of a 16-ounce (473.12-milliliter) bottle of shampoo left after she completed all her appointments for the day, she had $\frac{1}{2}$ of the bottle remaining. The fraction $\frac{1}{2}$ is a whole lot easier to work with than $\frac{8}{16}$ is.

QUESTION 3: How should Juan, in the example above, simplify the fraction $\frac{8}{32}$ to create an easier number to work with?

ANSWER: **STEP 1:** To make this fraction useable and understandable, we must find the greatest common factor. To determine this, we must list all the factors of 8 and 32. This can be done through the use of division or multiplication. We could say what two numbers multiplied together equal 8, or we could ask what number can 8 be divided by?

STEP 2: Find the largest factor of the numerator and the denominator.

1, 2, 4, and 8   factors of the numerator 8

1, 2, 4, 8, 16, and 32   factors of the denominator 32

STEP 3: Determine the greatest common factor (GCF).

8   the greatest common factor of 8 and 32

STEP 4: Divide the numerator and the denominator by the greatest common factor.

$$\frac{8}{32} \div 8$$

or

$$8 \div 8 = 1$$
$$32 \div 8 = 4$$

Juan has $\frac{1}{4}$ of the bottle of shampoo remaining.

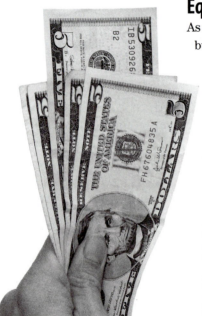

Equivalent Fractions

As defined earlier, an equivalent fraction is when two fractions look different but have the same value and are obtained when we either multiply or divide the numerator and the denominator of a fraction by the same number. Fractions, like money, can look different but have the same value. For example, four $5 bills are equal to one $20 bill, but they look very different.

A fraction has many equivalent fractions that have the same value but look different. An equivalent fraction can be found by either multiplying or dividing the numerator and the denominator by the same number.

Why are equivalent fractions important to the salon or spa professional? When completing an inventory list, you will come across a variety of products—in this case, let's discuss conditioner. Your salon or spa may have bottles of conditioner in a variety of sizes all around the salon. For example, at the backbar you may have a gallon or liter size of conditioner for use on clients when they are being shampooed and prepared for services, but at the cutting station you may have a 4-ounce (118.28-milliliters) bottle of conditioner that you keep there to discuss and educate clients with and finally, in the reception area, you may have a whole shelf of 16-ounce (473.12-milliliter) and 32-ounce (946.24-milliliter) bottles of the same conditioner for sale. If you are completing a salon inventory, you may need to know how much of that conditioner you have on hand in the salon in *total*—that means without regard for what size bottle it is in. To do that efficiently, you must not only determine how much is in each bottle of conditioner (determine the fractions), but you need to find a way to make those fractions equivalent (equal to one another) in order to get a total.

Let's start out with a simple equation and build up from there.

SHOW ME HOW

QUESTION 1: Mary has $\frac{1}{2}$ of a bottle of conditioner left on the backbar after using it on a week's worth of clients. What other fractions can represent the amount of conditioner that is left?

ANSWER: **STEP 1:** Determine what the denominator must be changed to.

Let's make the denominator 16. Where did the 16 come from? We could have just made it up, because we can change the denominator to any multiple of 2 that we choose so long as we multiply or divide the numerator and the denominator by the same number. In this case though, 16 has special significance because it is the total volume of the bottle of conditioner—16 ounces (473.12 milliliters).

STEP 2: Multiply the numerator and the denominator by the same number to achieve the desired result. To do this, we have to multiply both the numerator and the denominator of $\frac{1}{2}$ by 8. Multiplying the numerator and the denominator by 8 allows us to change the denominator to 16 and create an equivalent fraction at the same time.

$$\frac{1 \times 8}{2 \times 8} =$$

STEP 3: Make the product of the numerator and the denominator your answer.

$$\frac{1 \times 8}{2 \times 8} = \frac{8}{16}$$

The fraction left in the bottle can also be expressed as $\frac{8}{16}$. This will come in handy later when you have to add together more fractions—like bottles of conditioner that are $\frac{3}{16}$ or $\frac{7}{16}$ full.

QUESTION 2: Today Mike used $\frac{2}{3}$ of a bag of clean, white terry towels. What other fractions can represent the amount of towels that Mike used?

ANSWER: **STEP 1:** Determine what the denominator needs to be changed to. In this case, because the towels are laundered and delivered back to the salon in bags of 12, let's make the denominator 12.

STEP 2: Multiply the numerator and the denominator by the same number to achieve the desired result. If the goal is to get the denominator to 12, then we have to multiply the current denominator (3) by 4 to get 12. So we multiply both the numerator and the denominator by 4.

$$\frac{2 \times 4}{3 \times 4}$$

STEP 3: Make the product in the numerator and the denominator your answer.

$$\frac{2 \times 4}{3 \times 4} = \frac{8}{12}$$

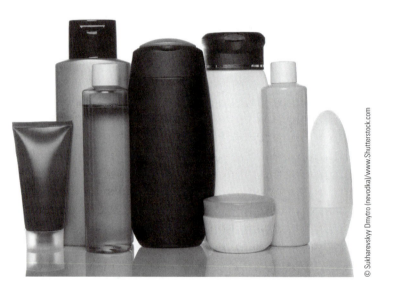

© Sukharevskyy Dmytro (nevodka)/www.Shutterstock.com

DID YOU KNOW? Do to the numerator what you do to the denominator of a fraction and then you will know that you have an equivalent fraction. Remember to always simplify or reduce a fraction when possible.

3–1 LET ME TRY

Simplify the following fractions.

1. $\frac{8}{20} =$ _____

2. $\frac{15}{35} =$ _____

3. $\frac{21}{28} =$ _____

Find equivalent fractions for the following fractions.

4. $\frac{1}{2} = $ _____

5. $\frac{3}{5} = $ _____

6. $\frac{2}{7} = $ _____

ADDING AND SUBTRACTING FRACTIONS

You have heard the old adage "You can't add apples and oranges," haven't you? It holds true in the mathematics world because, for example, we can't add $\frac{3}{4}$ and $\frac{2}{3}$ because they do not have the same denominators. When adding or subtracting fractions, two different numbers could have the same value, but we can only add or subtract things that are the same types of objects. When adding or subtracting fractions, the bottom numbers have to be the same to complete the equation.

If you have two jars of relaxer, and one is $\frac{2}{3}$ full and the other is $\frac{1}{4}$ full, how much relaxer do you have in total? How do we add $\frac{2}{3}$ and $\frac{1}{4}$?

When adding fractions we encounter two types of situations—*like denominator fractions* and *unlike denominator fractions*. You have **like denominator fractions** when the bottom numbers of the two fractions are the same. You have **unlike denominator fractions** when the bottom numbers of the two fractions are not the same.

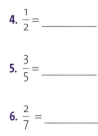 **DID YOU KNOW?**   Fractions can only be added when the bottom numbers (denominators) are the same.

Adding and Subtracting Like Denominator Fractions
Let's take a look at how to add and subtract like denominator fractions.

SHOW ME HOW

QUESTION 1:   Savannah used $\frac{2}{7}$ jar of monomer powder performing services for her nail clients on Monday and $\frac{3}{7}$ of a jar of monomer powder performing services for her nail clients on Tuesday. How much monomer powder did Savannah use altogether?

ANSWER: **STEP 1:** Make sure that the denominators are alike.

$\frac{2}{7}$ and $\frac{3}{7}$ amount of monomer powder used each day

$7 = 7$ denominator of both fractions

STEP 2: Add the numerators together.

2	numerator from the fraction for Monday
+ 3	numerator from the fraction for Tuesday
= 5	total of both numerators

STEP 3: Use the sum of the numerators over the denominator to create your answer.

$$\frac{2+3}{7} = \frac{5}{7}$$

Savannah used $\frac{5}{7}$ of a jar of monomer powder to service her nail clients between the two days.

QUESTION 2: Marshall has one tube of 5N in the haircolor dispensary until his delivery arrives tomorrow. He used $\frac{1}{5}$ of the tube on Tuesday morning when formulating Mrs. Jakard's haircolor formula and $\frac{2}{5}$ of the tube of 5N on Tuesday afternoon when formulating Deidra Sunder's haircolor. How much of the tube of 5N did Marshall use in total? Is there any 5N left?

ANSWER: **STEP 1:** Make sure that the denominators are alike.

$$\frac{1}{5} + \frac{2}{5} \qquad \text{amount of haircolor used}$$

$$5 = 5 \qquad \text{denominator of both fractions}$$

STEP 2: Add the numerators together.

$$\begin{array}{rl} 1 & \text{numerator of the fraction from Tuesday morning} \\ +\,2 & \text{numerator of the fraction from Tuesday afternoon} \\ \hline =\,3 & \text{total of both numerators} \end{array}$$

STEP 3: Use the sum of the numerators over the denominator to create your answer.

$$\frac{1+2}{5} = \frac{3}{5}$$

Marshall used $\frac{3}{5}$ of the tube of 5N and he has $\frac{2}{5}$ of the tube left over.

QUESTION 3: Amy started the day with $\frac{5}{7}$ of a bottle of shampoo that had been opened the day before, and by noon she had used $\frac{4}{7}$ of the bottle. How much shampoo did Amy have left in the bottle?

ANSWER: **STEP 1:** Make sure that the denominators are alike.

$$\frac{5}{7} \text{ and } \frac{4}{7} \qquad \text{amount of shampoo used over two days}$$

$$7 = 7 \qquad \text{denominator of both fractions}$$

STEP 2: Subtract the numerators.

$$5 - 4 = 1$$

STEP 3: Use the difference of the numerators over the denominator to create your answer.

$$\frac{5-4}{7} = \frac{1}{7}$$

Amy has $\frac{1}{7}$ of the bottle of shampoo remaining.

QUESTION 4: Andrew had $\frac{8}{11}$ of a bottle of massage oil that was left from the day before; he used $\frac{3}{11}$ of the oil at the start of today. How much oil will be left in the bottle if Andrew does not use any more massage oil for the remainder of the day?

ANSWER: **STEP 1:** Make sure that the denominators are alike.

$$\frac{8}{11} - \frac{3}{11} \qquad \text{amount of massage oil used today}$$

$$11 = 11 \qquad \text{denominator of both fractions}$$

STEP 2: Subtract the numerators.

$8 - 3 = 5$

STEP 3: Use the difference of the numerators over the denominator to create your answer.

$$\frac{8-3}{11} = \frac{5}{11}$$

Andrew has $\frac{5}{11}$ of the bottle of massage oil left.

Adding and Subtracting Unlike Denominator Fractions

Now it is time to explore how to add and subtract fractions when their denominators are not the same. This is a situation you will likely encounter often in the salon and spa because, while managing inventory, as noted earlier in the chapter, different materials can come in different-sized containers.

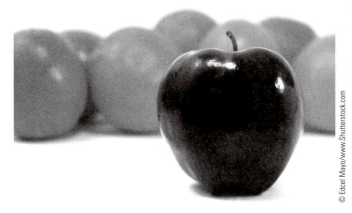

© Edcel Mayo/www.Shutterstock.com

To accomplish this, you have to find the **least common multiple (LCM)**, which is the smallest answer in a set of multiples that two denominators share in common. The word *multiple* comes from the same root word as *multiply*. The **LCM** is used to create equivalent values of a fraction for purposes of adding and subtracting fractions that we are not otherwise able to add or subtract.

SHOW ME HOW

QUESTION 1: When preparing a disinfectant solution, Jim filled $\frac{1}{3}$ of a spray bottle with concentrated disinfectant, and diluted it by filling $\frac{2}{5}$ of the same bottle with water. How much liquid did the spray bottle contain after dilution?

ANSWER: **STEP 1:** Find the least common multiple.

The bottom numbers of these fractions are not the same—$\frac{1}{3}$ and $\frac{2}{5}$—so we must find a way to make them the same. We can do this by finding the least common multiple (denominator) of the fractions. So if we multiply or count by 3 and 5, we will find the multiples of 3 and 5.

3, 6, 9, 12, 15, 18, 21, 24, 27, 30, etc.   multiples of 3

5, 10, 15, 20, 25, 30, 35, 40, 45, etc.   multiples of 5

15   least common multiple (LCM) of 3 and 5

STEP 2: Use the LCM to find the equivalent fractions.

So we must change both bottom numbers to 15. Now remember, whatever we do to the bottom we must also do to the top so that we will always have an equivalent fraction.

$$\frac{1}{3} = \frac{1 \times 5}{3 \times 5} = \frac{5}{15}$$ multiply both numbers by 5 in order to get the LCM of 15

$$\frac{2}{5} = \frac{2 \times 3}{5 \times 3} = \frac{6}{15}$$ multiply both numbers by 3 in order to get the LCM of 15

STEP 3: Add the equivalent fractions.

Now we are ready to add. We add the two equivalent fractions instead of the original fractions because the equivalent fractions have like denominators.

$$\frac{5}{15} + \frac{6}{15} = \frac{5 + 6}{15} = \frac{11}{15}$$

The bottle will be $\frac{11}{15}$ full.

QUESTION 2: Angela was tidying the color mixing bar area and pulled out several partially used bottles of developer. Before placing an order for additional developer, Angela needs to know how much developer the salon has in total.

ANSWER: **STEP 1:** Find the Least Common Multiple.

    7, 14, 21, 28, 35, 42, 49, 56, 63, 70   least common multiples of 7

    4, 8, 12, 16, 20, 24, 28, 32, 36, 40   least common multiples of 4

LCM: 28

STEP 2: Use the LCM to find the equivalent fractions—add the two equivalent fractions instead of the original fractions because the equivalent fractions have the same denominators.

$$\frac{1 \times 4}{7 \times 4} = \frac{4}{28}$$ multiply both numbers by 4 in order to get the LCM of 28

and

$$\frac{1 \times 7}{4 \times 7} = \frac{7}{28}$$ multiply both numbers by 7 in order to get the LCM of 28

STEP 3: Add the equivalent fractions.

$$\frac{4}{28} + \frac{7}{28} = \frac{4 + 7}{28} = \frac{11}{28}$$

After adding up the two partially used bottles of developer, the salon has $\frac{11}{28}$ of developer.

QUESTION 3: Latisha had $\frac{3}{4}$ of a jar of relaxer left over from yesterday, and she used $\frac{1}{6}$ of the jar of relaxer today. How much relaxer does Latisha still have left in the jar?

ANSWER: **STEP 1:** Find the LCM.

    4, 8, 12, 16, 20, 24, 28, 32, 36, 40   least common multiples of 4

    6, 12, 18, 24, 30, 36, 42, 48, 54, 60   least common multiples of 6

LCM: 12

STEP 2: Use the LCM to find the equivalent fractions.

$$\frac{3 \times 3}{4 \times 3} = \frac{9}{12}$$ multiply both numbers by 3 in order to get the LCM of 12

and

$$\frac{1 \times 2}{6 \times 2} = \frac{2}{12}$$ multiply both numbers by 2 in order to get the LCM of 12

STEP 3: Subtract the equivalent fractions.

$$\frac{9}{12} - \frac{2}{12} = \frac{9 - 2}{12} = \frac{7}{12}$$

Latisha's jar of relaxer is $\frac{7}{12}$ full.

QUESTION 4: Sandra had $\frac{5}{6}$ of a tube of haircolor remaining on Friday. On Saturday morning, she used $\frac{1}{7}$ of the tube of haircolor. How much haircolor is left in the tube?

ANSWER: **STEP 1:** Find the LCM.

6, 12, 18, 24, 30, 36, 42, 48, 54, 60   least common multiples of 6

7, 14, 21, 28, 35, 42, 49, 56, 63, 70   least common multiples of 7

42   the least common multiple of 6 and 7

STEP 2: Use the LCM to find the equivalent fractions.

$$\frac{5}{6} = \frac{5 \times 7}{6 \times 7} = \frac{35}{42}$$ multiply both numbers by 7 in order to get the LCM of 42

and

$$\frac{1}{7} = \frac{1 \times 6}{7 \times 6} = \frac{6}{42}$$ multiply both numbers by 6 in order to get the LCM of 42

STEP 3: Subtract the equivalent fractions.

$$\frac{35}{42} - \frac{6}{42} = \frac{35 - 6}{42} = \frac{29}{42}$$

Sandra has $\frac{29}{42}$ of haircolor left in the tube.

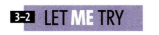 **LET ME TRY**

1. $\dfrac{3}{5} + \dfrac{2}{5} =$ _____

2. $\dfrac{6}{11} - \dfrac{5}{11} =$ _____

3. $\dfrac{3}{5} + \dfrac{1}{3} =$ _____

4. $\dfrac{5}{6} - \dfrac{3}{4} =$ _____

MULTIPLYING AND DIVIDING FRACTIONS

Although inventory counting and planning can be a lot of hard work, it is easier when you know the mathematical processes that enable you to count and tally effectively. So far you have added and subtracted fractions, and the more you practice, the better and quicker at it you will become.

Now we are going to move forward and discuss multiplying and dividing fractions. There will be situations when multiplying or dividing fractions will be a more efficient use of your time, and once you try it, you will see that it too is easy and saves you time.

In preparation for multiplying and dividing fractions, there are a few terms and concepts you need to be familiar with. For example, multiplying a group of prime numbers together to come up with a product is called **prime factorization**. A prime number has only two factors—1 and itself. The number 2 is the only even prime number because all of the other even numbers can be divided by 1 itself and the number 2.

When multiplying fractions, the fraction needs to be simplified or reduced using one of two methods: the *greatest common factor method* or the *cross-canceling method*.

The **greatest common factor method** is a way of simplifying a fraction by finding the common factors or multipliers of two numbers. For example, how do we simplify $\frac{12}{30}$? We begin by determining the multipliers of each number:

1, 2, 3, 4, 6, 12   the multipliers of 12
1, 2, 3, 5, 6, 10, 15, 30   the multipliers of 30

Now, you can see that the greatest common factor is 6, which means 6 is the largest number we can divide both 12 and 30 by and still get an even number:

$12 \div 6 = 2$
$30 \div 6 = 5$

When a numerator and a denominator cancel each other out through division by a common factor, it is called **cross-canceling**. Cross-canceling is a simplifying process. We can save time and work by using the cross-canceling method when multiplying fractions. Here is how it works. Let's say that we want to multiply $\frac{1}{4}$ by $\frac{2}{3}$; 2 and 4 can be cross-canceled or, in other words, divided be the factor 2. We get to the reduced answer more easily by reducing these numbers *before* we multiply, so the equation looks like this: $\frac{1}{2} \times \frac{1}{3}$. By using the cross-canceling method, we avoid dealing with large digits and then having to reduce our answer.

Remember that in division, a factor is a number that can divide into another number, creating an answer that is a whole number. A factor is also part of a multiplication problem. A factor is the two numbers that are multiplied together to create the product.

The inverting of a fraction or, in other words, reversing the top and bottom numbers of the fraction is called its **reciprocal**. An example of this is that the reciprocal of $\frac{3}{4}$ is $\frac{4}{3}$.

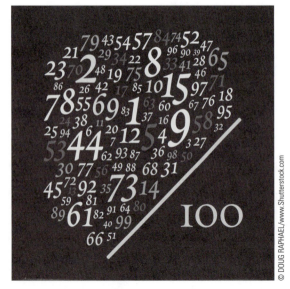

Multiplying Fractions with the Greatest Common Factor Method

Remember that the greatest common factor method is a way of simplifying a fraction by finding the common factors or multipliers of two numbers.

SHOW ME HOW

QUESTION 1: Ally needs to use $\frac{5}{10}$ of a container of neutralizer that is $\frac{2}{6}$ full to neutralize a relaxer on Lilly Kate's hair. How much neutralizer will Ally use?

ANSWER: STEP 1: Multiply the numerators together and then multiply the denominators together.

$\frac{2}{6}$ the amount of neutralizer in the container Ally started with

$\times \frac{5}{10}$ the amount of neutralizer in the container that Ally will use on Lilly Kate's hair

$2 \times 5 = 10$

$6 \times 10 = 60$

$= \frac{10}{60}$

STEP 2: Search for a common factor between the numerator and the denominator. The answer must be simplified or reduced. Remember to always simplify fractions to their lowest terms.

1, 2, 5, 10	multipliers of 10
1, 2, 3, 4, 5, 6, 10, 15, 20, 30, 60	multipliers if 60
10	the greatest common factor of 10 and 60

STEP 3: Simplify the fraction to its lowest term by dividing both the numerator and denominator by 10.

Which equals $\frac{10}{60} = \frac{10 \div 10}{60 \div 10} = \frac{1}{6}$

Ally used $\frac{1}{6}$ of a container of neutralizer on Lilly Kate's hair.

QUESTION 2: Sara has the responsibility to cleanup the salon tonight after the salon closes. Sara decides to use $\frac{2}{7}$ of $\frac{3}{5}$ of a liquid floor-cleaning solution to mop the salon's floor. How much of the cleaner did Sara use?

ANSWER: STEP 1: Multiply the numerators together and then multiply the denominators together.

$\frac{3 \times 2}{5 \times 7} = \frac{6}{35}$

STEP 2: Search for a common factor between the numerators and the denominators.

1, 2, 3, 6   multipliers of 6

1, 5, 7, 35   multipliers of 35

The numerator 6 and the denominator 35 do not share a common factor. Because the fraction cannot be simplified any further, the answer is $\frac{6}{35}$.

Sara used $\frac{6}{35}$ of a liquid floor-cleaning solution to mop the salon's floor.

Multiplying Fractions with the Cross-Canceling Method

Remember that cross-canceling is when a numerator and a denominator cancel each other out through division by a common factor. Cross-canceling is another simplifying process. We can save time and work by using the cross-canceling method when multiplying fractions.

Here we use the cross-canceling method to solve the same problems in the previous section, "Multiplying Fractions with the Greatest Common Factor Method."

SHOW ME HOW

QUESTION 1: Ally needs to use $\frac{5}{10}$ of a container of neutralizer that is $\frac{2}{6}$ full to neutralize a relaxer on Lilly Kate's hair. How much neutralizer will Ally use?

ANSWER: **STEP 1:** Look for numbers in the numerator and denominator that both share a common factor.

$$\frac{2}{6} \times \frac{5}{10}$$

The numbers 2 and 10 share a common factor, which is 2.

STEP 2: Divide the numerator and the denominator by the greatest common factor.

$$\frac{2 \div 2}{6} \times \frac{5}{10 \div 2} = \frac{1}{6} \times \frac{5}{5}$$

Now, because $\frac{5}{5}$ can be further simplified, do so before proceeding.

$$\frac{1}{6} \times \frac{5 \div 5}{5 \div 5} = \frac{1}{6} \times \frac{1}{1}$$

STEP 3: Multiply the numerator and the denominator in the new fractions together.

$$\frac{1}{6} \times \frac{1}{1} = \frac{1}{6}$$

Ally used $\frac{1}{6}$ of a container of neutralizer on Lilly Kate's hair.

QUESTION 2: Sara has the responsibility to cleanup the salon tonight after the salon closes. Sara decides to use $\frac{2}{7}$ of $\frac{3}{5}$ of a liquid floor-cleaning solution to mop the salon's floor. How much of the cleaner did Sara use?

ANSWER: **STEP 1:** Look for numbers in the numerator and denominator that both share a common factor for $\frac{2}{7}$ and $\frac{3}{5}$. Remember, in order to cross-cancel we have to have one number on the top of either fraction that shares a common factor of one of the numbers that is on the bottom of either fraction. The numbers do not have to be vertically on the top and bottom; they could also be diagonally on the top and bottom. We discover that in this case the numbers do not share a common factor. So we are unable to use the cross-canceling method to solve this equation.

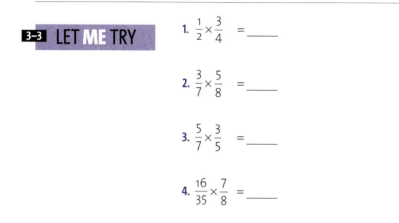

3-3 LET ME TRY

1. $\frac{1}{2} \times \frac{3}{4}$ = _____

2. $\frac{3}{7} \times \frac{5}{8}$ = _____

3. $\frac{5}{7} \times \frac{3}{5}$ = _____

4. $\frac{16}{35} \times \frac{7}{8}$ = _____

Did you remember to simplify and/or cross-cancel?

Dividing Fractions Without Cross-Canceling

In order to divide fractions, we must remember this very important rule of thumb: We *never* divide fractions; instead we must change the division problem into a multiplication problem. As long as we have a change to offset a change, we will be fine. Remember: *Change, Change* equals the same. So what shall we change? Well, we have a special rule for this, too. The special rule is that we always change the last fraction to its reciprocal. Let's take a look at all of this action.

SHOW ME HOW

QUESTION 1: Jasmine had $\frac{5}{9}$ of a bottle of peroxide remaining on Friday. If she used $\frac{1}{9}$ of the $\frac{5}{9}$ on each client's hair on Saturday, how many clients could Jasmine service with the remaining peroxide?

ANSWER: $\frac{5}{9} \div \frac{1}{9}$

STEP 1: Change the operation from division to multiplication, and change the fraction following the operation to its reciprocal.

change $\frac{5}{9} \div \frac{1}{9}$

to

$\frac{5}{9} \times \frac{9}{1}$

Now we are ready to solve the problem.

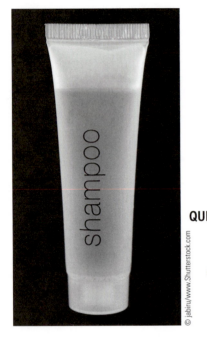
© jabiru/www.Shutterstock.com

STEP 2: Multiply the numerators together, and then multiply the denominators together.

$$\frac{5}{9} \times \frac{9}{1} = \frac{45}{9}$$

STEP 3: Simplify the fraction to the lowest term by dividing 45 and 9 by the GCF (which is 9).

$$\frac{45 \div 9}{9 \div 9} = \frac{5}{1} = 5$$

Jasmine has enough peroxide to service 5 clients.

QUESTION 2: Bob had $\frac{3}{4}$ of a bottle of shampoo. If he used $\frac{3}{16}$ of the $\frac{3}{4}$ that was left in the bottle on each client's hair, how many clients could Bob shampoo?

ANSWER: **STEP 1:** Change the operation from division to multiplication, and change the fraction following the operation to its reciprocal.

$$\text{change } \frac{3}{4} \div \frac{3}{16} \text{ to } \frac{3}{4} \times \frac{16}{3}$$

STEP 2: Multiply the numerators together, and then multiply the denominators together.

$$\frac{3}{4} \times \frac{16}{3} = \frac{48}{12}$$

STEP 3: Simplify the fraction to the lowest term by dividing 12 and 48 by the GCF (which is 12).

$$\frac{48 \div 12}{12 \div 12} = \frac{4}{1} = 4$$

Bob can shampoo 4 clients with the remainder of shampoo in the bottle.

Dividing Fractions with Cross-Canceling

Remember that cross-canceling is when a numerator and a denominator cancel each other out through division by a common factor. Cross-canceling is another simplifying process. We can save time and work by using the cross-canceling method when dividing fractions, as long as we remember one simple rule: Never ever cross-cancel before you change your problem to a multiplication operation.

Let's revisit the previous examples using the cross-canceling method of simplifying the answer this time.

SHOW ME HOW

QUESTION 1: Jasmine had $\frac{5}{9}$ of a bottle of peroxide remaining on Friday. If she used $\frac{1}{9}$ of the $\frac{5}{9}$ on each client's hair on Saturday, how many clients could Jasmine service with the remaining peroxide?

ANSWER: **STEP 1:** Change the operation from division to multiplication, and change the fraction following the operation to its reciprocal.

$$\frac{5}{9} \div \frac{1}{9} \text{ becomes } \frac{5}{9} \times \frac{9}{1}$$

STEP 2: Look for numbers in the numerator and denominator that both share a common factor.

The common factor in this case is 9.

$$\frac{5}{9 \div 9} \times \frac{9 \div 9}{1} = \frac{5}{1} \times \frac{1}{1}$$

STEP 3: Multiply the numerators together, then multiply the denominators together and simplify when possible.

$$\times = \frac{5}{1} = 5$$

Jasmine has enough peroxide to service 5 clients.

QUESTION 2: Bob had $\frac{3}{4}$ of a bottle of shampoo. If he used $\frac{3}{16}$ of the $\frac{3}{4}$ that was left in the bottle on each client's hair, how many clients could Bob shampoo?

ANSWER: **STEP 1:** Change the operation from division to multiplication, and change the fraction following the operation to its reciprocal.

$$\frac{3}{4} \div \frac{3}{16} \text{ becomes } \frac{3}{4} \times \frac{16}{3}$$

STEP 2: Look for numbers in the numerator and denominator that both share a common factor (in this case there are two, both 3 and 4 can be used).

$$\frac{3 \div 3}{4 \div 4} = \frac{16 \div 4}{3 \div 3} = \frac{1}{1} \times \frac{4}{1}$$

STEP 3: Multiply the numerators together, then multiply the denominators together and simplify when possible.

$$\frac{1}{1} \times \frac{4}{1} = \frac{4}{1} = 4$$

Bob can shampoo 4 clients with the remainder of shampoo in the bottle.

3–4 LET ME TRY

1. $\frac{3}{7} \div \frac{4}{7} = $ _____

2. $\frac{5}{8} \div \frac{15}{40} = $ _____

3. $\frac{21}{25} \div \frac{14}{15} = $ _____

4. $\frac{32}{45} \div \frac{24}{30} = $ _____

1. What is a fraction? Give three examples of fractions.

2. How are fractions simplified? Why is this useful in inventory management?

3. Describe what an equivalent fraction is and give three examples.

4. Describe the process for adding fractions with like denominators.

5. Describe the process for subtracting fractions with like denominators.

6. Describe the process for adding fractions with unlike denominators.

7. Describe the process for subtracting fractions with unlike denominators.

8. Define the greatest common factor method and explain how it is used in multiplying and dividing fractions.

9. What is the cross-canceling method, and how is it used in multiplying fractions?

10. Describe how to divide fractions without using the cross-canceling method.

11. Explain how to divide fractions using the cross-canceling method.

CHAPTER 4

Purchasing Principles

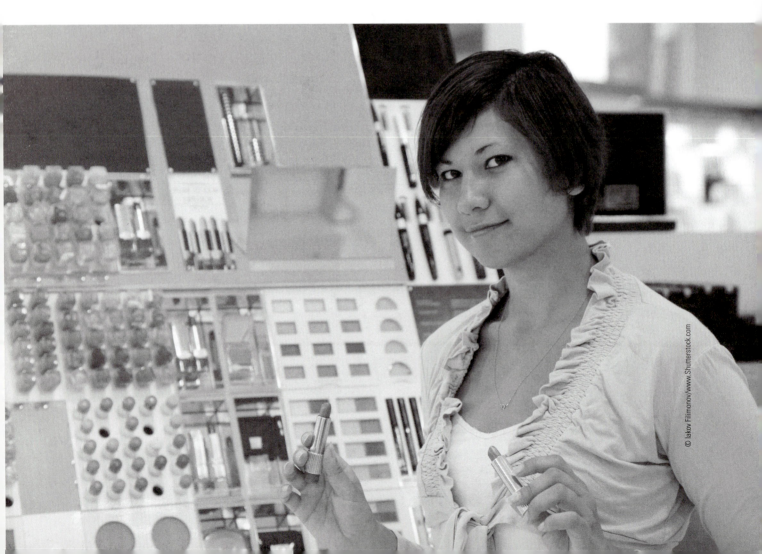

- Decimals
- Converting Fractions, Decimals, and Percentages
- Exponents
- Order of Operations

LEARNING OBJECTIVES

After completing this chapter, you will be able to:

1. Identify and define a decimal.

2. Add and subtract decimals.

3. Multiply and divide decimals.

4. Convert a fraction to a decimal.

5. Convert a decimal to a percentage.

6. Recognize and understand exponents.

7. Multiply exponents to simplify problem-solving.

8. Recite and use the proper order of operations for all mathematical processes.

KEY TERMS

- absolute value bars
- base
- brackets
- converting
- decimals
- digits
- exponential form
- exponents
- first rule
- mathematical logic
- order of operation
- parentheses
- PEMDAS
- place value
- power
- product rule
- radical sign
- rounded number
- standard form
- zero rule

I N THE PREVIOUS CHAPTER, WE EXPLORED HOW TO MANAGE AND COUNT inventory using fractions. We learned that no matter the size of the container or the amount in the container, we could add, subtract, multiply, and divide to help us keep track of inventory and plan for product usage. Now, we are going to explore other mathematical concepts that help to make purchasing of products and goods easier to understand.

DECIMALS

In Chapter 3, we learned how to use fractions to account for supplies that had been partly used; now we are going to take a look at another way of counting parts of the whole—decimals. A piece or part of an item can be represented by a fraction *or* a decimal, and every fraction has an equivalent decimal value. Sometimes it is easier to use decimals (such as when you are reviewing the invoice from your beauty supplier or when looking at your bank statement), and sometimes it is easier to use fractions (such as when you are counting the partially used bottles of shampoo on the salon's backbar).

Decimals are always used in the discussion and review of money. For example, you would never see an invoice that says you owe $6\frac{3}{4}$ dollars, would you? The invoice would say you owe $6.75.

Decimals are like fractions because they represent a piece or a part of a whole number. Decimals are best understood by relating them to money. The numbers to the right of the decimal represent a piece or a part of a whole dollar. All decimals have equivalent fraction and percent values.

Digits are the numerical symbols that make up a number. The digits by themselves do not have a numerical value except to identify the total of certain place value. An example of a digit would be 3 in the number 234.56. The 3 does not have a value by itself, but it does identify that there are 3 *tens* in the "tens" place value. A digit's **place value** is the value each digit holds in a specific location in reference to the decimal point in a number. All numbers have a decimal point—some are visible (2.56) and others are invisible (3). For example, in the number 2.56 the 2 represents a whole number: 2. The 5 represents 5 "tenths" of a number, and 6 represents 6 "hundredths" of a number.

The following chart, called the *Place Value Chart*, will help you to see what value each place represents. Note that whole numbers begin at the value titled "*ones*," and decimals are to the right of the ones.

© pixelfabrik/www.Shutterstock.com

© Milady, a part of Cengage Learning.

One millionths	Hundred thousands	Ten thousands	One thousands	Hundreds	Tens	Ones	Decimal	Tenths	Hundredths	Thousandths	Ten thousandths	Hundred thousandths	One millionths
							•						

When working with numbers and inventory, or when purchasing inventory, it may be necessary for you to convert one form of a number to another. **Converting** is when the appearance of a number is changed so that the number looks different but still has the same value. An example of this concept is $\frac{1}{4}$. $\frac{1}{4} = 0.25 = 25\%$. All fractions, decimals, whole numbers, and percents can be converted into each other.

© almagami almagami/www.Shutterstock.com

SHOW ME HOW

Use the place value chart on the previous page to answer the following questions:

QUESTION 1: What is the place value of the digit 8 in the number 234.578?

ANSWER: Determine which side of the decimal point the number is on. In the number 234.578, 8 is the third number from the decimal point. If you count three to the right of the *ones* on the chart, you find that the place value of 8 is *thousandths*.

QUESTION 2: What is the place value of the digit 6 in the number 345.654?

ANSWER: Determine which side of the decimal point the number is on. In the number 345.654, 6 is the first number after the decimal point. If you count one to the right of the *ones* on the chart, you find that the place value of 6 is *tenths*.

QUESTION 3: What is the place value of the digit 3 in the number 312.6245?

ANSWER: Determine which side of the decimal point the number is on. In the number 312.6245, 3 is the third number on the left of the decimal point. If you count three to the left of the *ones* on the chart, you find that the place value of 3 is *hundreds*.

4-1 LET ME TRY

1. What is the place value of the digit 7 in the number 173.456?

2. What is the place value of the digit 6 in the number 183.256?

3. What is the place value of the digit 9 in the number .00295?

Adding and Subtracting Decimals

Adding or subtracting decimals requires the lining up of the decimals over each other and simply adding or subtracting the numbers. Adding and subtracting decimals have the same rules as other addition and subtraction. Let's try a few equations so you can get used to working with decimals.

SHOW ME HOW

QUESTION 1: Andrea's supplies for the month of January cost $315.76, and her supplies for the month of February cost $258.62. What was the total cost of the supplies for both months?

ANSWER: **STEP 1:** Make sure the problem is written vertically, not horizontally, and line up the decimal points, one over the other.

$$\begin{array}{r} \$\ 315.76 \\ +\ \$258.62 \\ \hline \end{array}$$

STEP 2: Add the digits, carry, and borrow when needed.

$$\begin{array}{r} \$\ 315.76 \\ +\ \$258.62 \\ \hline =\ \$574.38 \end{array}$$

Andrea's supplies for the two months cost $574.38.

QUESTION 2: Charlie paid $325 for a nail class he wanted to take at the local beauty supply house, and he paid $32.45 for the required supplies to take the class. How much did Charlie spend to take the class?

ANSWER: **STEP 1:** Make sure the problem is written vertically, not horizontally, and line the decimals up in the problem, one over the other. Note, if there is a place value where there is nothing, then a zero may be placed into that place value. Zero is the digit that represents nothing.

$$\begin{array}{r} \$325.00 \\ +\ \$\ \ 32.45 \\ \hline \end{array}$$

STEP 2: Add the digits, carry, and borrow when needed.

$$\begin{array}{r} \$325.00 \\ +\ \$\ \ 32.45 \\ \hline \$357.45 \end{array}$$

Charlie spent $357.45 to take the class.

QUESTION 3: Rhonda was debating between purchasing two different relaxers. One relaxer cost $32.58 and the other cost $28. How much money will Rhonda save by purchasing the less expensive relaxer?

ANSWER: **STEP 1:** Make sure the problem is written vertically, not horizontally, and line the decimals up in the problem, one over the other.

$$\begin{array}{r} \$32.58 \\ -\ \$28.00 \\ \hline \end{array}$$

STEP 2: Subtract the digits, carry, and borrow when needed.

$32.58
− $28.00
$ 4.58

Rhonda will save $4.58 by purchasing the less expensive of the two products.

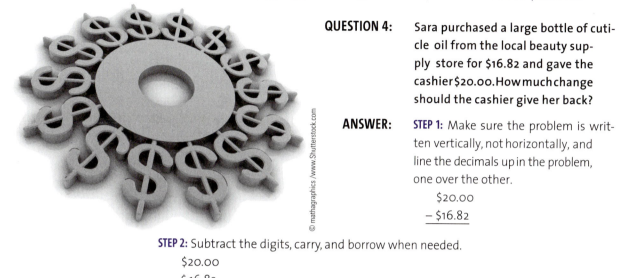

QUESTION 4: Sara purchased a large bottle of cuticle oil from the local beauty supply store for $16.82 and gave the cashier $20.00. How much change should the cashier give her back?

ANSWER: **STEP 1:** Make sure the problem is written vertically, not horizontally, and line the decimals up in the problem, one over the other.

$20.00
− $16.82

STEP 2: Subtract the digits, carry, and borrow when needed.

$20.00
− $ 16.82
$ 3.18

Sara should receive $3.18 back in change from the cashier.

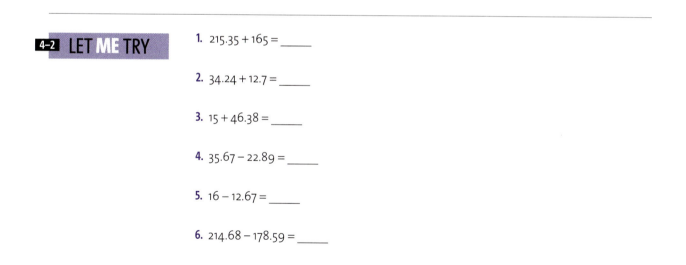

4–2 LET ME TRY

1. 215.35 + 165 = _____

2. 34.24 + 12.7 = _____

3. 15 + 46.38 = _____

4. 35.67 − 22.89 = _____

5. 16 − 12.67 = _____

6. 214.68 − 178.59 = _____

Multiplying and Dividing Decimals

There are times when you need to multiply and divide decimals. For example, while managing your inventory, you realize that you need to purchase supplies. Specifically, you notice that the spa has 15 pedicures booked for the upcoming week, but you do not have any pedicure slippers on hand. You call your supplier and find out that pedicure slippers cost $.59 each, and you need to determine how much it will cost you to order 15 for the week. What do you do? You need to multiply!

Multiplying decimals is accomplished in two steps—first you multiply the numbers without regard for the decimal points, then you count how many numbers in the problem are to the right of the decimal point, and then place that many numbers to the right of the decimal in the answer. In the cases we are going to be looking at, we take the multiplying and dividing decimals one step further—we also apply mathematical logic.

Mathematical logic is the science of using correct reasoning. When we *reason*, we make an argument for or against something based on certain assumptions or premises.

For example, consider the following *inference* (the act of passing from one proposition, statement, or judgment considered as true to another whose truth is believed to follow from that of the former):

Some salons and spas generate their owner great wealth.

Anything that generates great wealth is a good investment.

Therefore, some salons and spas are good investments.

In the following section, you are asked to apply logic, or reasoning, to your final answer. For example, in the case of money, we know that it is not logical for something to cost $.6524609, so we know that we *round* the final answer to $.65, or sixty-five cents. A **rounded number** is an approximate number rather than an exact number.

SHOW ME HOW

QUESTION 1: Cathy needs to order 15 pairs of pedicure slippers to accommodate the 15 pedicures the spa has booked that week. Each pair of pedicure slippers costs $.59. How much do the 15 pairs of slippers cost?

ANSWER: **STEP 1:** Make sure the problem is written vertically, not horizontally.

$$\begin{array}{r} \$.59 \\ \times\, 12 \\ \hline \end{array}$$

STEP 2: Multiply the numbers together, ignoring the decimals.

$$\begin{array}{r} \$.59 \\ \times\, 12 \\ \hline = 708 \end{array}$$

STEP 3: Determine where the decimal should go in the final answer by counting how many digits come after the decimal points in the problem.

$.59	2 numbers are to the right of the decimal point
× 12	0 numbers are to the right of the decimal point
= $7.08	therefore, 2 numbers go after the decimal point in the final number

STEP 4: Apply logic to the final answer.

$7.08 is an acceptable answer for describing money. There should only be two numbers to the right of the decimal point when describing money. Therefore we do not have to do anything else. Cathy paid $7.08 for 15 pairs of pedicure slippers.

QUESTION 2: Tim purchased 6 tubes of haircolor for $8.45 per tube. Tim used 4.5 tubes of haircolor. How much was the total price of the 4.5 tubes of haircolor that Tim used?

ANSWER: STEP 1: Make sure the problem is written vertically, not horizontally.

$$\begin{array}{r} \$8.45 \\ \times\, 4.5 \\ \hline \end{array}$$

STEP 2: Multiply the numbers together, ignoring the decimals.

$$\begin{array}{r} \$8.45 \\ \times\, 4.5 \\ \hline = \$38025 \end{array}$$

STEP 3: Determine where the decimal should go in the final answer by counting how many digits come after the decimal points in the problem.

$$\begin{array}{r} \$8.45 \\ \times\, 4.5 \\ \hline = \$38.025 \end{array}$$ 2 numbers are to the right of the decimal point
1 number is to the right of the decimal point
therefore, 3 numbers go after the decimal point in the final number

STEP 4: Apply logic to the final answer.

$38.025 is not an acceptable answer for describing money. There should only be two numbers to the right of the decimal when describing money. Therefore, we will have to drop the 5 and round the 2 up to the next value, which is 3. We round up if the number following the 2 is 5 or greater. In this case, it is, so our final answer is $38.03. The total cost of the of the 4.5 tubes of haircolor that Tim used is $38.03.

QUESTION 2: Robin purchased 12 quarts (11.35 liters) of 20-volume clear developer for $1.89 each. How much did Robin pay for all 12 quarts (11.35 liters) of 20-volume clear developer?

ANSWER: STEP 1: Make sure the problem is written vertically not horizontally.

$$\begin{array}{r} \$1.89 \\ \times\, 12 \\ \hline \end{array}$$

STEP 2: Multiply the numbers together, ignoring the decimals.

$$\begin{array}{r} \$1.89 \\ \times\, 12 \\ \hline = 2268 \end{array}$$

STEP 3: Determine where the decimal should go in the final answer.

$$\begin{array}{r} \$1.39 \\ \times\, 12 \\ \hline = \$22.68 \end{array}$$ 2 numbers are to the right of the decimal point
o numbers are to the right of the decimal point
therefore, 2 numbers go after the decimal point in the final number

STEP 4: Apply logic to the final math answer.

$22.68 is an acceptable answer for describing money. There should only be two numbers to the right of the decimal point when describing money. Therefore, we do not have to do anything else. Robin paid $22.68 for all 12 quarts (11.35 liters) of 20-volume clear developer.

Now, let's assume that you are doing some cost analysis, trying to determine the price of the products you use on a per client basis. For example, you bought

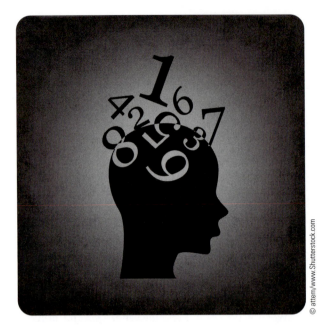

a 6-ounce (168-gram) tube of haircolor for $4.95. You used 2 ounces (56 grams) of it in your last color formulation, and now you want to know how much that 2 ounces (56 grams) cost. What do you do? You divide and you multiply!

Dividing decimals requires moving the decimal in the divisor, which is the number that is doing the dividing. The decimal should be placed to the right of the last digit in the divisor. Because the decimal is to be moved in the divisor, then the decimal must be moved in the dividend, which is the number that is being divided. The decimal in the divisor and the dividend must be moved the same amount of decimal places. After moving the decimals, the dividend has to be divided by the divisor.

SHOW ME HOW

QUESTION 1: Johnny bought a 6.85-ounce (191.8-gram) tube of haircolor for $4.95 and used 2 ounces (56 grams) of it in his last color formulation. What was the cost of the 2 ounces (56 grams) Johnny used?

ANSWER: **STEP 1:** First, we must find out how much each ounce of the haircolor cost. Set the problem up as a division problem.

$4.95 ÷ 6.85

STEP 2: Move the decimal to the right the same amount of places in both numbers until it is no longer in the divisor (6.85). In this case, you move the decimal 2 places to the right.

$4.95 ÷ 6.85
= 495 ÷ 685

STEP 3: Divide normally.

495 ÷ 685 = .7226

STEP 4: Apply logic to the answer.

.7226 is not an acceptable answer for describing money. There should be only two numbers to the right of the decimal when describing money to account for the dimes and pennies. If you count two digits to the right of the decimal point, the answer is $.72 per ounce.

STEP 5: Multiply the cost per ounce by the number of ounces used.

$.72	cost per ounce of haircolor
× 2	number of ounces used
= $1.44	cost of using 2 ounces of that tube of haircolor

QUESTION 2: Andy purchased a 2.05-ounce (57.4-gram) tube of haircolor for $4.55. How much did Andy pay for 1 ounce (28 grams) of the haircolor?

ANSWER: **STEP 1:** First, we must find out how much each ounce of the haircolor cost. Set the problem up as a division problem.

$4.51 ÷ 2.05

STEP 2: Move the decimal to the right the same amount of places in both numbers until it is no longer in the divisor (2.05). In this case, you move the decimal 2 places to the right.

$4.51 ÷ 2.05
= 451 ÷ 205

STEP 3: Divide normally.

451 ÷ 205 = 2.2

STEP 4: Apply logic to the final math answer.

$2.2 is not an acceptable answer for describing money. There should be two numbers to the right of the decimal when describing money to account for the dimes and pennies. Because there are no pennies, we add a zero to the right of the dimes place value because zero represents nothing. Our final answer is $2.20 per ounce. Andy paid $2.20 for 1 ounce of the haircolor.

QUESTION 3: Erin is reviewing her sales invoice for some bottles of shampoo she purchased. The total cost is $51.12 and each bottle of shampoo cost $6.39. How many bottles of shampoo did Erin purchase?

ANSWER: **STEP 1:** Set the problem up as a division problem.

$51.12 ÷ $6.39

STEP 2: Move the decimal to the right the same amount of places in both numbers until it is no longer in the divisor ($6.39). In this case, move the decimal 2 places to the right.

5112 ÷ 639

STEP 3: Divide as usual.

5112 ÷ 639 = 8

STEP 4: Apply logic to the final math answer.

The number 8 is an acceptable answer for describing objects. Therefore, our final answer is that 8 bottles of shampoo were purchased.

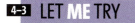 **4-3 LET ME TRY**

1. 32.56 × 12 = _____

2. 23.45 × 3.45 = _____

3. 2.345 × 100 = _____

4. 61.52 ÷ 15.38 = _____

5. 12.36 ÷ .02 = _____

6. 512.6 ÷ 2.13 = _____

CONVERTING FRACTIONS, DECIMALS, AND PERCENTAGES

We can use decimals instead of fractions if we convert the fraction to a decimal. Fractions, decimals, and percentages are three different ways we can represent the value of a piece or part of a whole number. Every decimal has an equivalent fraction and percent that have the same value, much like one dollar can be represented by paper currency, coins, or a check. The more ways we can represent a value, the stronger our math skills become. Let's look at how we can convert decimals, fractions, and percentages.

Sometimes you need to change the way a fraction looks to make it look like a decimal so you can proceed with a calculation.

Converting a Fraction to a Decimal

For example, someone may tell you that she has have $\frac{1}{2}$ a dollar, and wants to spend it on an item. $\frac{1}{2}$ is a fraction, but when money is discussed, used, and calculated, it is calculated using decimals. So how do you convert a $\frac{1}{2}$ to a decimal?

SHOW ME HOW

QUESTION 1: Hannah has $\frac{1}{2}$ a dollar—how much money does she actually have?

ANSWER: **STEP 1:** Divide the numerator by the denominator.

$1 \div 2 = .5$

STEP 2: Apply logic to the answer.

.5 of a $1.00 is $.50, or fifty cents.

QUESTION 2: Marcel used $\frac{5}{8}$ of a tube of haircolor. What decimal represents the amount of haircolor Marcel used?

ANSWER: **STEP 1:** Divide the numerator by the denominator.

$5 \div 8 = .625$

STEP 2: Apply logic to the answer.

Because this number goes beyond two digits after the decimal place, we round the number to .63. Because the third number is a 5, we round up. So, Marcel used .63 of the tube of haircolor.

Converting a Decimal to a Percentage

There may also be times when you want or need to convert a decimal to a percentage, for ease of calculation and/or understanding.

QUESTION 1: How would you convert .75 to a percentage?

ANSWER: **STEP 1:** Move the decimal 2 places to the right, which makes the decimal invisible if there no other digits to the right of the decimal.

.75 becomes 75. when the decimal is moved

STEP 2: Add a percentage sign.

75%

QUESTION 2: Mark has decided to become $\frac{1}{3}$ of a partnership in a salon his friends are opening. They need $100,000 start-up money. What percentage of the $100,000 is Mark expected to invest?

ANSWER: **STEP 1:** Divide the numerator by the denominator

$1 \div 3 = .3333333$

STEP 2: To determine the percentage Mark needs to contribute, move the decimal 2 places to the right, which makes the decimal invisible if there no other digits to the right of the decimal.

.33 = 33%

Mark needs to invest 33% of the $100,000 start-up money.

QUESTION 3: Anne just received her paycheck. She sees that, in addition to her regular hourly wage, she has received monies for her retail sales. Anne knows that she gets 15% commission on all of her retail sales and that her retail sales totaled $136 this week. How much money should she have received for her retail sales?

ANSWER: **STEP 1:** Multiply total retail sales by the percentage paid.

$136 \times 15\% = x$

STEP 2: Move the decimal point two places to complete the multiplication.

$136 \times .15 = 20.4$

Apply logic to the final answer. Ann should have received $20.40 in retail commissions in this paycheck.

EXPONENTS

Can you solve this problem? There is a bus taking cosmetology students to a trade show. There are 7 students in the bus. Each student has 7 backpacks. In each backpack, there are 7 curling irons. For every curling iron there are 7 flat irons. How many people and objects are on the bus?

This is definitely a math problem that can be solved with multiplication, but there is so much multiplication that it will be a very big problem and extremely difficult to solve. Fortunately, this type of multiplication problem can be made shorter and easier to solve by using exponents.

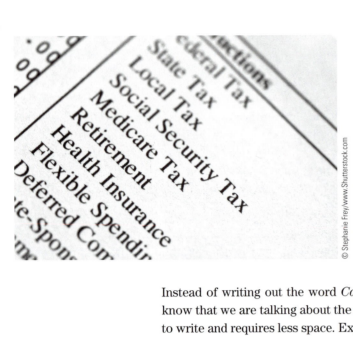

Exponents are special types of multiplication problems whereby the same number is multiplied by itself as many times as stated by the power. An exponent contains a **base**, the number that is to be multiplied, and a **power**, also known as *superscript*, the number that determines how many times the base is to be multiplied by its self.

Here is an example of an exponent; it looks like this: 8^3. The 8 is the *base* and the 3 is the *power*. The problem should be read as 8 to the 3rd power and is solved by multiplying 8 by 8 three times: $8^3 = 8 \times 8 \times 8 = 512$.

Exponents are similar to abbreviations. Instead of writing out the word *California* we simply write *CA*. Both ways let us know that we are talking about the state of California, but the abbreviation is faster to write and requires less space. Exponents save time and space.

Why is it important for beauty professionals to know about exponents? Well, imagine this: You purchase 3 cases of shampoo that have 3 bottles of shampoo in each case, and you make this purchase 3 times a year. You could use the exponent principle to determine how much shampoo you buy in a year.

To solve this problem, you use the **exponential form**, writing the problem as an exponent. If we are trying to solve the shampoo question, and we write the problem in the exponential form, it looks like this: $3 \times 3 \times 3 = 3^3$.

If we decide not to use the exponential form but rather to write the problem in the usual way, we expect to see a multiplication problem—$3 \times 3 \times 3$—which is called the **standard form**.

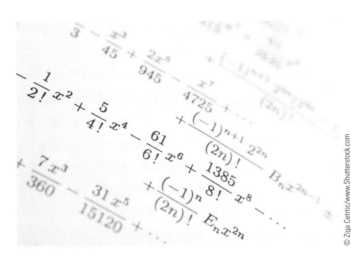

Using exponents especially comes in handy when purchasing product and determining costs. And there are additional rules for when we are adding or multiplying more than one exponent. For example, the **product rule** states that any time we multiply exponents together that have the same base, we simply add the powers together. An example of this concept is $2^3 \times 2^2 = 2^{3+2} = 2^5 = 32$. Remember, this works as long as the base is the same.

Here are a few more concepts to be aware of before we start using the concepts to solve everyday purchasing issues. The **zero rule** states that anytime we raise a base to the zero power, the answer is 1. An example of this concept is $5^0 = 1$

The first rule states that anytime we raise a base to the first power, the answer is the base. An example of this concept is $5^1 = 5$.

Now it is time to see exponents in action.

SHOW ME HOW

QUESTION 1: Steve purchased 4 cases of peroxide that had 4 bottles of peroxide in each case 4 times a year. How many bottles of peroxide did Steve purchase a year?

ANSWER: **STEP 1:** Determine whether there is a set of the same numbers that have to be multiplied together.

4 cases of shampoo @ 4 bottles per case @ 4 times a year =
$4 \times 4 \times 4$

STEP 2: Identify the base and identify the power or superscript.

4   the base number
3   the power or superscript number

STEP 3: Write the exponent that represents the multiplication problem.

$4^3 = 4 \times 4 \times 4$

STEP 4: Solve the multiplication problem. Remember, exponents are about saving time and space, but we still have to perform the same operations no matter how the problem is written.

$4^3 = 64$

Steve purchased 64 bottles of peroxide each year.

QUESTION 2: Ernie purchased 5 cases of conditioner that have 5 bottles of conditioner in each case, for $5 per bottle for the last 5 months of the year. What was the total amount of money that Ernie paid for all of the conditioners for the last 5 months of the year?

ANSWER: **STEP 1:** Determine whether there are sets of the same set of numbers that have to be multiplied together.

$5 each apiece @ 5 bottles per case @ 5 cases @ 5 months
$5 \times 5 \times 5 \times 5 =$

STEP 2: Identify the base and identify the power or superscript.

5   the base number
4   the power or superscript number

STEP 3: Write the exponent that represents the multiplication problem.

$5^4 = 5 \times 5 \times 5 \times 5$

STEP 4: Solve the multiplication problem.

$5^4 = 625$

Ernie paid $625 for all of the conditioner he bought in the last five months of the year.

QUESTION 3: Nancy purchased 4 cases of shampoo that had 4 bottles of shampoo in each case and 6 cases of shampoo that had 6 bottles of shampoo in each case. How much shampoo did Nancy purchase all together?

ANSWER: **STEP 1:** Determine whether there are sets of the same numbers that have to be multiplied together.

4 cases @ 4 bottles per case and 6 cases @ 6 bottles per case
$4 \times 4 + 6 \times 6$

STEP 2: Identify the base and identify the power or superscript.

    4 and 6   the base numbers

       2   the power or superscript number

STEP 3: Write the exponent that represents the multiplication problem.

$4^2 + 6^2 = 4 \times 4 + 6 \times 6$

STEP 4: Solve the multiplication and addition problem.

$4^2 + 6^2 = 4 \times 4 = 16 + 6 \times 6 = 36$

$16 + 36 = 52$

Nancy purchased 52 bottles of shampoo altogether.

QUESTION 4:   Donna purchased 5 cases of haircolor that had 5 tubes in each case for \$5 per tube, and she purchased the same amount every 2 weeks for 2 months. How much did all the haircolor cost Donna?

ANSWER: **STEP 1:** Determine whether there are sets of the same numbers that have to be multiplied together.

    \$5 a tube @ 5 tubes per case @ 5 cases @ 2 Weeks @ 2 Months

    $5 \times 5 \times 5 \times 2 \times 2$

STEP 2: Identify the base and identify the power or superscript.

    5 and 2   the base numbers

    3 and 2   the power or superscript numbers

STEP 3: Write the exponent that represents the multiplication problem.

    $5^3 \times 2^2 = 5 \times 5 \times 5 \times 2 \times 2$

STEP 4: Solve the multiplication problem.

    $5^3 \times 2^2 = 125 \times 4 = 500$

Donna spent \$500 on all of the haircolor she purchased.

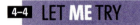 **LET ME TRY**

For the following equations, give the exponential form of the problem.

1. $5 \times 5 \times 5 \times 5 \times 5 \times 5 \times 5 = $ _____

2. $3 \times 3 \times 3 \times 3 = $ _____

3. $6 \times 6 = $ _____

For the following equations, give the standard form of the problem.

4. $2^4 = $ _____

5. $8^2 = $ _____

6. $3^2 \times 3^3 = $ _____

ORDER OF OPERATIONS

In the beauty business, as in mathematics, there is a certain order to things; certain things need to be done first in order for the operation to come out correctly. For example, you would never apply neutralizer to a head full of perm rods *before* you applied the waving lotion, or primer to the nails *after* you applied the monomer powder and the polymer liquid, would you? Of course you wouldn't—if you did that, the operation or procedure would not be correctly completed.

Well, mathematics is exactly the same way. When calculating, especially discounts and purchases, the order with which you perform the operations is important if you want to arrive at an accurate total.

Order of operation states that when there are different operations in a problem, they must be completed in a specific order. There are several operations that may be required to complete a problem. They include: performing operations in parentheses and/or other grouping symbols, exponents, multiplication, division, addition, and subtraction. One easy way to remember the order of what gets done first is to use the acronym **PEMDAS**. PEMDAS is an acronym that was created by taking the first letter of each of the operations in the order that they should be done.

Order of Operation

P Parentheses
E Exponents
M Multiplication
D Division
A Addition
S Subtraction

Parentheses are grouping symbols that allow us to group things that are alike, or similar to each other, together so that they can be combined into one value prior to performing any other operations. An example of this concept is adding all the sales together, because they are alike, prior to multiplying them by the sales tax rate: $(30 + 40 + 40) \times 7\% = (110) \times .07 = \$7.70$.

Brackets are grouping symbols like parentheses that allow us to group things that are alike, or similar to each other, together so that they can be combined into one value prior to performing any other operations. An example of this concept would be $[30 + (40 + 40)] \times 7\% = [30 + 80] \times .07 = [110] \times .07 = \$7.70$.

Absolute value bars are grouping symbols that measure a numbers distance from zero. Absolute values are always positive values. There cannot be a negative distance from zero. An example of this concept is $|3 - 8| = |-5| = 5$, that is, that the absolute value of -5 is 5 units from zero.

Radical signs are grouping symbols that determine the root of a number. An example of this concept is $\sqrt{10 - 1} = \sqrt{9} = 3$. That is to say that $3 \times 3 = 9$.

Remember that exponents are a way of notating a special type of multiplication problem in order to save time and space. Exponents should be performed after all grouping symbols such as parentheses and brackets have been addressed.

Multiplication and division should be performed from *left to right*. Multiplication and division have a special relationship so much so that they are treated the same when addressing many rules.

Addition and subtraction should also be performed from *left to right*. Addition and subtraction, like multiplication and division, have a special relationship so much so that they are treated the same when addressing many rules.

Let's take a look at an example of an equation that requires knowledge and use of the PEMDAS principle:

$$(3 + 5) \times 2^2 - 6 + 4$$

STEP 1: Do what is in the parentheses first.
$(3 + 5) = 8$, so now the equation looks like this: $8 \times 2^2 - 6 + 4$

STEP 2: Multiply the exponents next.
$2 \times 2 = 4$, so now the equation looks like this: $8 \times 4 - 6 + 4$

STEP 3: Now complete any additional multiplication.
$8 \times 4 = 32$, so now the equation looks like this: $32 - 6 + 4$

STEP 4: Next, complete any addition.
$6 + 4 = 10$, so now the equation looks like this: $32 - 10 =$

STEP 5: Finally, complete any subtraction.
$32 - 10 = 22$. The answer to the equation is 22.

Ready to see PEMDAS in action? Here are some great examples taken from typical situations you may find yourself in.

SHOW ME HOW

QUESTION 1: Lyla purchased 3 cases of perms containing 3 boxes per case, for $3 each. The supplier agrees to give Lyla a 10% discount on the purchase. However, Lyla must pay a 7% sales tax on the purchase of the supplies. What is the total Lyla has to pay for the perms?

ANSWER: **STEP 1:** Write the problem as an equation.

$[3^3$	sales
$-(3^3 \times 10\%)]$	discount
$+(3^3 \times 7\%)$	sales tax

STEP 2: Change percentages to decimals.

$[3^3$
$-(3^3 \times .10)]$
$+(3^3 \times .07)$

STEP 3: Perform inner grouping of parentheses in brackets from left to right (in other words complete the operations of any numbers that are in parentheses inside of brackets).

$[3^3 - (3^3 \times .10)] + (3^3 \times .07)$ becomes
$[3^3 - (27 \times .10)] + (3^3 \times .07)$ becomes
$[3^3 - (2.7)] + (3^3 \times .07)$

STEP 4: Perform operations of the outer grouping, completing what is in the brackets and the parentheses from left to right.

$[3^3 - (2.7)] + (3^3 \times .07)$ becomes

$[27 - (2.7)] + (3^3 \times .07)$ becomes

$[24.3] + (27 \times .07)$ becomes

$[24.3] + (1.89)$

STEP 5: Perform the addition, making sure to line up the decimals correctly.

$$
\begin{aligned}
24.3 \\
+\,1.89 \\
\hline
=\,26.19
\end{aligned}
$$

Lyla paid a total of $26.19 for the perms she bought.

QUESTION 2: Maggie purchased 3 liters of shampoo for $10 each, a can of hair spray that was $6, and 1 gallon of conditioner for $15. Maggie is told by her DSC that the hair spray is on sale for 20% off the regular price. Once she adds the 7% sales tax to her purchase, what is the total of Maggie's cost?

ANSWER: **STEP 1:** Write the problem as an equation.

$(3 \times 10 + 6 + 15)$ sales

$-(6 \times 20\%)$ discount

$+[(3 \times 10 + 6 + 15) \times 7\%]$ sales tax

STEP 2: Change percentages to decimals

$(3 \times 10 + 6 + 15) - (6 \times .20) + [(3 \times 10 + 6 + 15) \times .07] = \text{Total}$

STEP 3: Perform inner grouping of parentheses in brackets from left to right (in other words complete the operations of any numbers that are in parentheses inside of brackets).

$(3 \times 10 + 6 + 15) - (6 \times .20) + [(30 + 6 + 15) \times .07]$ becomes

$(3 \times 10 + 6 + 15) - (6 \times .20) + [51 \times .07]$

STEP 4: Perform operations of the outer grouping completing what is in the brackets and the parentheses from left to right.

$(30 + 6 + 15) - (6 \times .20) + [51 \times .07]$ becomes

$(51) - (6 \times .20) + [51 \times .07]$ becomes

$(51) - (1.2) + 3.57$ becomes

$49.8 + 3.57$

STEP 5: Perform the addition, making sure to line up the decimals correctly.

$$
\begin{aligned}
49.8 \\
+\,3.57 \\
\hline
\$53.37
\end{aligned}
$$

Solve these problems. Remember to follow the correct order of operations.

1. $4 \times 3^2 - 3 =$ _____

2. $(10 + 20) \div 5 =$ _____

3. $10 + (20 \div 5) =$ _____

4. $8 \times 3 + 2 \times 5 =$ _____

5. $5 + (2 \times 2 + 4)^2 =$ _____

6. $5 \times (3^2 - 7) =$ _____

1. What is a decimal and what does it look like?

2. Add 534.87 and 45.09.

3. Subtract 34.76 from 100.43.

4. Multiply 32.12 by 18.

5. Divide 564.98 by 98.36.

6. Convert the fraction $\frac{5}{21}$ to a decimal.

7. Convert the decimal .643 to a percentage.

8. Define exponents and explain how they are used.

9. Give three examples of exponents, and write a mathematical equation that explains each.

10. Multiply the following exponents: 6^9, 12^3, 3^6.

11. What is PEMDAS and what does it stand for?

Pricing Products and Services and Determining Profit

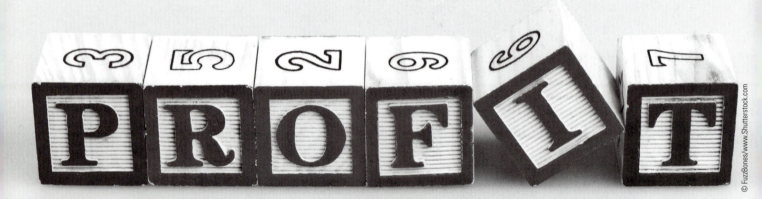

CHAPTER OUTLINE

- Pricing and Promotion
- The Mathematics of Pricing and Promotion

LEARNING OBJECTIVES

After completing this chapter, you will be able to:

1. Define a promotion and describe why they are used in business.

2. Determine a product pricing strategy and calculate sales price.

3. Determine a service pricing strategy and explain the components of such a strategy.

4. Understand the purpose and use of a target profit margin.

5. Define and describe profit.

6. Identify the Formula Table and understand its use.

7. Write a mathematical expression.

8. Simplify a mathematical expression.

KEY TERMS

- constant
- equation
- evaluating
- formula
- gross profit
- like terms

- linear equation
- linear inequalities
- math expression
- net profit
- profit
- profit margin

- promotions
- simplify
- term
- unlike terms
- variable

SO FAR IN THIS TEXT, WE HAVE REVIEWED BASIC MATHEMATICAL OPERATIONS; appointment planning and scheduling clients; and inventory management and purchasing principle. Now it is time to take a good look at pricing products and services and all that comes along with this aspect of the salon and spa business.

It would be easy to simply say, "I do facials, and so for the rest of my career I will perform the same 50-minute facial on every client, and I will always charge $70 for it." It would be simple, but not terribly realistic! Especially when the costs for products and supplies you use might go up; your rent and other expenses could increase; or maybe competition comes into the area so that you have to create interest-generating special pricing. These are just some of the reasons why beauty professionals need to carefully plan out their pricing and profit strategies.

In this chapter, we will explore all of the figures you should know and use when calculating your product and service pricing, and how to determine your profits once you know the costs of performing services and doing business.

PRICING AND PROMOTION

Heather wants to offer specials that would increase business to her nail salon, but she does not want to lose money doing it, so she needs to know the cost of running the special before she starts. First, Heather needs to come up with a formula or a mathematical expression that defines the problem in mathematical terms.

Let's take a look at the Heather's idea more carefully, starting with *Heather wants to offer specials that would increase business to her nail salon …* ; the word *specials* in this sentence implies that Heather is considering offering discounts—or value-added **promotions**, the furtherance of the acceptance and sale of merchandise through advertising, publicity, or discounting—to get more clients into her nail salon.

The second part of that sentence reads … *but she does not want to lose money doing it, so she needs to know the cost of running the special before she starts.* Heather realizes that running the special may bring more business into the salon; but it could cost more than usual to offer and will probably cut into her profits, so she must have a good handle on, and knowledge of, the costs involved, before jumping into a promotion.

Salon and spa professionals frequently find themselves in the same situation as Heather. For whatever reason—business is slow, appointments are scarce, or product/retail sales are sluggish—an automatic reaction is to "run a special."

Product and service promotions are perfectly legitimate ways of increasing traffic to the salon and exposing your business to new clients or to clients who have been absent for a long time. But before introducing a promotion, you need to know the true costs for your salon or spa.

© Arcady/www.Shutterstock.com

Before we begin, we will review some basic pricing and profit assumptions that are frequently present in the salon and spa world:

- When pricing retail products for sale in the salon, most businesses double *their* purchase price to create their sales price, rounding up to the nearest figure. So, for example, if you purchase a bottle of nail polish for $3.09, and double the price, it would be sold for $6.25 (rounding up to the nearest figure). The sales price is a 100% increase over the purchase price.

- A salon or spa must have a good, clear handle on the costs associated with each service it offers. These costs can include products used in the performance of the service, supplies used in the performance of the service, overhead, employee commission or salary for performing the service, and any proposed discount or promotion.

Generally a salon needs to make a *target profit margin* of 30% to 50% on every procedure, service, and treatment. The **profit margin** is the bare minimum below which, or the extreme limit beyond which, something becomes impossible or is no longer desirable. **Profit** is the excess of the selling price of goods after their cost has been subtracted and can be defined further in two ways: as gross profit and net profit. **Gross profit** is simply the difference between sales and costs of sales, meaning product usage. **Net profit** is the revenue left over after the cost of the service (products used) and expenses (such as overhead, advertising, etc.) are subtracted from the sales. So, for example, if it costs the salon $34 to cover all of the costs mentioned above for a haircolor service ($9 for products and supplies needed to perform the service, $5 for overhead, and $20 employee commission or salary for performing the service = $34), it needs to offer the service to clients for anywhere from $44 to $51 to achieve a 30% to 50% target profit margin. The selling price of the service is computed by taking the cost of the performing the service—$34—and multiplying it by 1.30 for a 30% profit margin, or 1.50 for a 50% profit margin.

If you do not know what your salon or spa's preferred profit margin is, then ask your manager or the owner. If you are the owner, you should consult with your accountant for help in determining your target profit percentages.

How does knowing this information help you? It helps because you know what the profit targets are before planning a promotion, sale, or discount program that may significantly eat into salon profits. This is not to say that there are not circumstances that make a promotion viable and worth running, even if it does not meet the financial targets of the salon. But is *does* mean that not every promotion can be allowed to miss those targets, or the salon will not show enough profit and could be in jeopardy of going out of business.

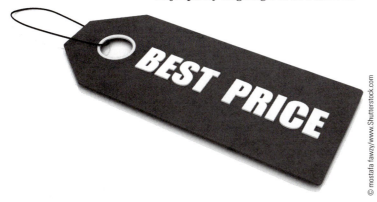

What are some of the circumstances that might make it wise to run a special, sale, or promotion that doesn't hit the preassigned profit targets?

- **Increased competition.** There may be a time when you find that the salon or spa is being competed against in a way it had not anticipated. For example, your spa has been the only one in a 5-mile radius for a number of years; then, only 1.5 miles away another spa opens. It is new and exciting, it offers some services that your spa does not, and it is targeting your spa's clientele. In this case, the management team at the spa may decide that a promotion or other special program is needed, and it is worth it to lose a little profit margin now to save clients in the long run.

- **Difficult economic climate.** Every economy has its ups and downs. When people have less money to spend or are trying to stretch their money farther because of economic conditions outside of their control, running specials and discount programs can be a way to retain more of your clients so that they do not leave your salon or spa altogether. This is a solid strategy for retaining clients in the hopes that when the economy turns around, these clients will continue to be loyal patrons of your business.

- **Increased cost of sales.** Sometimes the price of the treatment and service products you use increases and, theoretically, you should increase your prices to cover these costs. However, it can be difficult to ask clients to pay increased prices for products and services more than once a year. It is wise to set a schedule for increasing your prices and to stick to it unless there is some significant economic disaster. Pick one date when each year new prices will go into effect, and increase prices at that time. When determining pricing increases, try to figure in current and future costs of sales increases, and always give clients time to prepare for the increase.

THE MATHEMATICS OF PRICING AND PROMOTION

Mathematics helps in determining a pricing and promotional strategy. A **linear equation** is an equation for a straight line. A linear equation describes a relationship in which the value of one of the variables depends on the value of the other variable. Linear equations usually have constants and must have simple variables. **Linear inequalities** use a symbol to compare two things in order to determine whether one side on an equation is either equal to, less than, or greater than the other. In Chapter 1, we discussed how mathematics uses equations to communicate meaning. But, when trying to determine whether to run a special, for example, some information may be missing that we need to know in order to determine whether to proceed. A letter or symbol is used to represent some unknown numerical value or values. This unknown value is called the **variable**. Problems in linear equations focus on finding the variable. Understanding linear equations broadens our understanding of mathematics as a language with practical applications.

Here are a few more terms to be aware of as you continue with this chapter:

- A **constant** is a numerical value that is fixed and does not change.

- A **term** is a number or the product of a number and a variable raised to a power, such as 3, 7, $5y$, or $6x$.

- **Like terms** have the same variables and powers or exponents, such as $3x$, $5x$, $6x$, and $7x$.

- Terms are called **unlike terms** if they have different variables or powers or exponents, such as 3, $3x$, $3x^2$, and $3y$.

- A **math expression**, also known as a *formula*, is a math statement that is meaningful. It is a collection of numbers, variables, signs, and operations, such as $3x + 7$.

- To **simplify** is a mathematical process that makes a math expression easier to understand or solve through the use of the order of operation (PEMDAS), the associative property, the commutative property, and the distributive property; an example of this is: $3x + 5x - 7 = 8x - 7$.

- A **formula**, also known as a *math expression*, is a math statement that defines a real-world problem in math terms (see Table 5–1).

- An **equation** is a math statement that defines two math expressions as being equal to each other, such as $3x + 7 = 2x - 5$.

When we replace variables with some known numerical values and then perform the order of operations, it is called **evaluating**. For example, If $x = 5$ and $y = 7$, then to evaluate $3x - 2y$ you would replace the letters with their appropriate values and the equation would look like this: $3(5) - 2(7) = 15 - 14$, or 1.

Here are a few terms we learned earlier in the text to remember for this chapter:

- The *associative property* is a mathematical property that allows the moving or removal of parentheses when working with addition or multiplication. For example: $(3x + 5) + 6 = 3x + (5 + 6)$ becomes $(3x + 5) + 6 = 3x + 11$.

- The *commutative property* is a mathematical property that allows the moving of numbers around the operations when working with addition or multiplication. For example: $5 + 3x + 6 = 3x + 5 + 6$ becomes $5 + 3x + 6 = 3x + 11$.

- And finally, the *distributive property* is a mathematical property that multiplies the term on the outside of the parentheses by every term on the inside of the parentheses. For example: $3(x + 6) = 3 \bullet x + 3 \bullet 6$ becomes $3(x + 6) = 3x + 18$.

Every problem and solution can be defined in two ways—with words or with numbers. A formula or mathematical expression is a numerical way of defining a problem. Its solution is the answer to the problem.

FORMULA TABLE

Real-World Problem	Variables Defined	Formula
Tax	P = price; R = tax rate; T = tax	$T = P \times R$
Discount	P = price; R = discount rate; D = discount	$D = P \times R$
Sales Price	P = price; T = tax; D = discount; S = sales price	$S = (P - D) + T$
Sales	P = price; Q = quantity sold; S = sales	$S = P \times Q$
Cost	P = price; Q = quantity purchased; C = cost	$C = P \times Q$
Gross Profit	S = sales; C = cost; G = gross profit	$G = S - C$
Net Profit	S = sales; C = cost; E = expenses; N = net profit	$N = S - (C + E)$

In the table below are a list of words and symbols that denote basic math operations—watch for them in your problem solving.

Addition	Subtraction	Multiplication	Division
Sum	Difference	Product	Quotient
Increase	Decrease	Times	Divided by
More than	Less than	Per (increase)	Per (decrease)
Plus	Minus	Twice	Ratio
+	−	$\times$, ( ), $\cdot$, $3x$, xy	$\div$, $\overline{)}$, Fraction bar

© Milady, a part of Cengage Learning.

Let's take a look at several rules we will follow in this chapter:

- The variable is typically the first letter in the problem or the item that the variable represents.
- We will use the fraction bar to denote division $\left(\frac{1}{1}\right)$.
- We never use the times table symbol ($\times$) to denote multiplication because it might be confused with the letter or variable X; instead we use this symbol: $\cdot$.
- Unknown values or numbers are represented by the letter x in italics. This letter reminds us that unknowns have to be replaced with a number.

Writing Mathematical Expressions

Now, we are going to read some problems and take a stab at translating them—using numbers and symbols—into mathematical expressions that can be evaluated and eventually solved. Use the word clues in the problem and Table 5–1 to aid you in writing out the mathematical expression.

QUESTION 1: Macy purchased an unknown number of bottles of nail polish for $4 per bottle and sold the nail polish for $7 per bottle. What mathematical expression represents Macy's gross profit?

ANSWER: **STEP 1:** Determine the variables and constants needed to create the math expression. The constants and variables are: Cost = $4, Sales = $7, Quantity = x.

STEP 2: Determine the operations involved.
Because gross profit can be found by subtracting the total cost from the total sale, subtraction is one operation. The other operation is multiplication because the word *per* denotes multiplication.

STEP 3: Organize the math statement into a meaningful collection of numbers, variables, and signs of operations.

Gross Profit	=	Sales − Cost
Gross Profit	=	Price × Quantity − Price × Quantity
Gross Profit	=	$\$7(x) \times \$4(x)$
Gross Profit	=	$7x - 4x$

The math expression is $7x - 4x$.

QUESTION 2 Amy purchased 8 bottles of nail polish remover and 4 bottles of foot cream. The cost of the nail polish remover and the cost of the foot cream were equal. What mathematical expression represents Amy's cost for both items?

ANSWER: **STEP 1:** Determine the variables and constants needed to create the math expression. The constants and variables are: Quantity of nail polish remover = 8, Quantity of foot cream = 4, Price = x.

STEP 2: Determine the operations involved.
Because cost can be found by multiplying the price by the quantity, one operation is multiplication and the other is addition.

STEP 3: Organize the math statement into a meaningful collection of numbers, variables, and signs of operations.

Cost	=	Nail Polish Remover	+	Foot Cream
Cost	=	Price × Quantity	+	Price × Quantity
Cost	=	$(x)8$	+	$(x)4$

commute the multiplication

Total Cost	=	$8x$	+	$4x$

The mathematical expression is $8x + 4x$ before simplifying.

QUESTION 3: Rikki sold an unknown number of bottles of shampoo plus 5 more bottles of shampoo for $6 per bottle. Rikki paid $38 for all of the bottles of shampoo. What mathematical expression best represents Rikki's total profit?

ANSWER: **STEP 1:** Determine the variables and constants needed to create the math expression. The variables and constants are: Quantity of bottles = 5, Quantity of other bottles = x, Price = $6, Cost = $38.

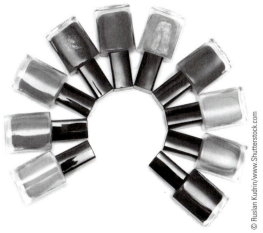

© Ruslan Kudrin/www.Shutterstock.com

STEP 2: Determine the operations involved. Because gross profit can be found by subtracting the total cost from the total sale, subtraction is one operation. The other operation is multiplication because the word *per* denotes multiplication when there is an increase.

STEP 3: Organize the math statement into a meaningful collection of numbers, variables, and signs of operations.

Gross profit	= Sales	− Cost
Gross profit	= Price × (Other Quantity + Quantity)	− Cost
Gross profit	= $\$6(x + 5)$	− $38

The math expression is $6(x + 5) - 38$ before simplifying.

5-1 LET ME TRY

1. Marie purchased an unknown number of bottles of cuticle softener for $5 per bottle and sold them for $8 per bottle. What mathematic expression represents Marie's total profit?

2. Frank purchased 7 jars of styling wax and 4 cans of hair spray for the same price. What mathematic expression represents Frank's total cost?

3. David sold an unknown number of bottles of top coat on Monday, and on Tuesday he sold 8 more bottles of top coat for $5 per bottle. David paid $33 for all of the bottles. What mathematical expression represents David's total profit?

Simplifying Mathematical Expressions

Remember that when we *simplify* in a mathematical process, we make the math expression easier to understand or solve through the use of the order of operation, associative property, commutative property, and distributive property. Let's get some practice simplifying the following.

DID YOU KNOW? Keep in mind that **PEMDAS** is an acronym that was created by taking the first letter of each of the operations in the order that they should be done.

Order of Operation

P Parentheses

E Exponents

M Multiplication

D Division

A Addition

S Subtraction

SHOW ME HOW

QUESTION 1: Use the distributive, associative, or order of operation to release the parentheses and combine like terms when possible in this equation:

$$3(x + 4)$$

ANSWER: **STEP 1:** Distribute the multiplication of 3 to every variable and number inside the parentheses over the addition operation.

$$3(x + 4) = 3 \cdot x + 3 \cdot 4$$

STEP 2: Follow the order of operation (PEMDAS) to simplify the problem.

$3 \cdot x + 3 \cdot 4 = 3x + 12$

$3(x + 4) = 3x + 12.$

QUESTION 2: Use the distributive, associative, or order of operation to release the parentheses and combine like terms when possible in this equation:

$2(x - 5) + 3x + 7$

ANSWER: **STEP 1:** Distribute the multiplication of 2 to every variable and number inside the parentheses over the subtraction operation.

$2(x - 5) + 3x + 7 = 2 \cdot x - 2 \cdot 5 + 3x + 7$

STEP 2: Follow the order of operation (PEMDAS) to simplify the problem.

$2 \cdot x - 2 \cdot 5 + 3x + 7 = 2x - 10 + 3x + 7$

STEP 3: Use the commutative property to move the terms around.

$2x - 10 + 3x + 7 = 2x + 3x + 7 - 10$

STEP 4: Simplify further by combining like terms. (**Note:** 7 − 10 is less than zero because we are taking away more than we have.)

$2x + 3x + 7 - 10 = 5x - 3$

$2(x - 5) + 3x + 7$ is equal to $5x - 3$.

QUESTION 3: Use the distributive, associative, or order of operation to release the parentheses and combine like terms when possible in this equation:

$5(2x + 3) + (-7x + 8)$

ANSWER: **STEP 1:** Distribute the multiplication of 5 to every variable and number inside the parentheses over the addition operation, and use the associative property to release the second set of parentheses.

$5(2x + 3) + (-7x + 8) = 5 \cdot 2x + 5 \cdot 3 + (-7x) + 8$

STEP 2: Follow the order of operation (PEMDAS) to simplify the problem.

$5 \cdot 2x + 5 \cdot 3 + (-7x) + 8 = 10x + 15 + (-7x) + 8$

STEP 3: Use the commutative property to move the terms around and then combine like terms.

$10x + 15 + (-7x) + 8 = 10x + (-7x) + 8 + 15$

STEP 4: Simplify further by combining like terms.

$10x + (-7x) + 8 + 15 = 3x + 23$

5-2 LET ME TRY

Translate these word problems into mathematical expressions, and use the Formula Table located on page 77 for guidance.

1. Jack purchased 6 bottles of nail polish for $3 each.
   a. What formula represents Jack's cost?

   b. Evaluate the formula if $Q = 6$, $P = \$3$

   c. What is Jack's cost for the 6 bottles of nail polish?

2. Janice charges $75 for a full set of gel nails but decides to give a 20% discount to attract new customers.
   a. What formula represents the sale price?

   b. If no tax is charged on the service, what is the formula?

   c. Evaluate the formula if P = $75 and R = .20.

   d. What is the discounted price for the service?

3. Annie sells a bottle of hand lotion for $5.69 plus sales tax, which is 7%.
   a. What formula represents the sales price?

   b. The bottle of hand lotion is sold at full price, with no discounts, what formula now resents the same price?

   c. Evaluate the formula if P = $5.69 and R = .07.

   d. What is the price for the bottle of hand lotion?

4. Marshall decides to run a special on pedicures. Marshall's spa normally charges $65 for a pedicure, but for the next week he decides to offer a 15% discount to attract new customers.
   a. What formula represents the net profit for this promotion?

   b. What is the sale price of the pedicure?

   c. Now assume that the costs and expenses involved in giving a pedicure are $1.50 for service products; $.50 for the clean linens used during the service; $27.62 representing a 50% commission to the pedicurist; $.76 for the cost of advertising the special; and finally, $3.25 for overhead, rent, electrical, etc. What is the total cost to the salon of offering this pedicure promotion?

   d. What is the net profit per pedicure that the salon will see once the pedicure promotion is underway?

1. What is a promotion? Why and when are promotions used in the salon and spa business?

2. Describe the standard product pricing strategy used in the salon and spa business. If products are purchased at the prices of $4.39, $2.98, $11.76, and $1.86, what would their sales price be?

3. Describe the standard service pricing strategy used in the salon and spa business, and name the costs that help determine the final price of a service.

4. What is a target profit margin, and how is it helpful when determining pricing and promotions?

5. Define and describe profit.

6. What is the Formula Table and how is it used?

7. Write a mathematical expression that best describes the following: Heather sells pumice stones for $4.85 each and the sales tax is 7%. What is the sales price of each pumice stone, including the sales tax?

8. Simplify this mathematical expression: $(3x + 5) + (2x + 7)$.

Meeting Financial Goals

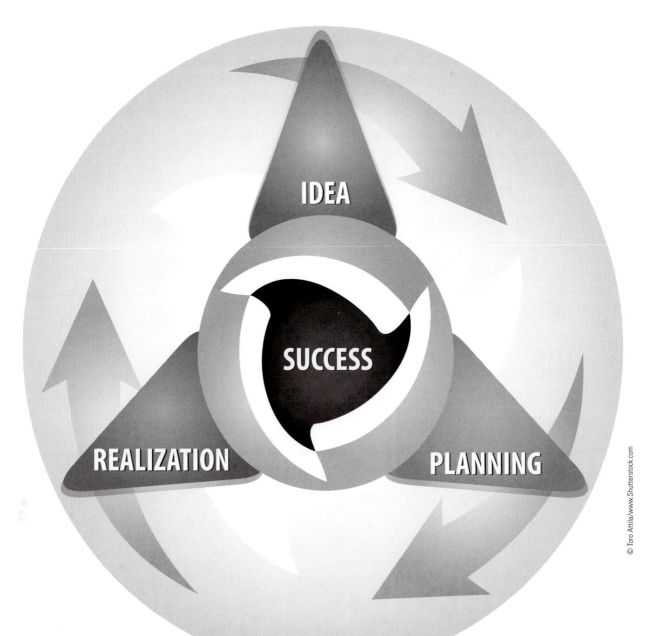

CHAPTER OUTLINE

- Service Planning and Profits
- Meeting and Exceeding Profit Goals
- Making Expense and Profit Projections
- Determining Minimum Expectations

LEARNING OBJECTIVES

After completing this chapter, you will be able to:

1. Understand the use of equations in profit planning and calculating.

2. Identify and understand the use of algorithms and the three types used in solving equations.

3. Describe the trial and error method of solving an equation.

4. Describe the addition method of solving an equation and when it is used.

5. Describe the multiplication method of solving an equation and when it is used.

KEY TERMS

- addition method
- algorithm
- boundary
- equations
- multiplication method
- solution
- trial and error method

ONE OF THE BIGGEST CHALLENGES IN RUNNING A BUSINESS IS MEETING ALL of its financial obligations. There is creating a service menu, which is of course all of the services the salon or spa will offer; then there is being able to purchase supplies for a reasonable price; hiring staff to perform these services, and then making enough money on the service to pay the staff person; and, ultimately, paying all of these costs and still having some profit left over to invest back into the business. Whew! That's a lot to think about. The good news is that mathematics can help you determine all of those figures which will make the meeting of these financial goals a little bit easier to understand and accomplish. This is the focus of this chapter.

SERVICE PLANNING AND PROFITS

In the previous chapter, we worked with mathematic expressions and formulas; now we can apply that knowledge to solve other problems. For example, Bob knows how much money he needs to earn and knows the price and cost of each item and service he provides, but does not know how many items or services he needs to provide in order to make the amount of money that he wants to earn. How would formulas solve a problem like that? This problem can be formulated as an *equation*.

Equations are mathematic statements that define two expressions as being equal to each other, such as in this example: $5 + $5 + $5 + $5 = $20.

We work with equations to find a **solution**, a numerical value that can replace a variable and cause the equation to be true. In other words, the right side will be equal to the left side after all of the operations are performed.

An **algorithm** is a mathematical process that is used to arrive at a desired outcome or solution. Some algorithms that might be used to solve equations are: the trial and error method, the addition method, and the multiplication method.

The **trial and error method** is an algorithm that requires the replacement of the variable with an *estimated* value until the correct value is found. The idea is to try to solve the equation with a new number each time until the correct value is found. Trial and error is a *guess and prove* method.

The **addition method** is an algorithm that requires the use of addition and subtraction to eliminate all values near the variable until the variable is isolated. The addition method is used when the equation involves addition or subtraction.

The **multiplication method** is an algorithm that requires the use of multiplication and division to eliminate all values near the variable until the variable is isolated. The multiplication method is used when the equation involves multiplication or division.

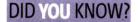

DID YOU KNOW? When using algorithms to solve equations, use the *CEI* rule:

- **C**onsolidate by combining like terms.
- **E**liminate by doing the same thing to both sides of the equation.
- **I**solate so that the value of the unknown will be known.

Let's take a look at some of these methods in action as we solve the following equations. Remember to refer to the Formula Table in Chapter 5 to determine your course of action.

SHOW ME HOW

QUESTION 1:   **A.** Heather charges $30 per manicure. She paid a total of $18 for supplies. After subtracting the cost of supplies, she made $162 on a day's worth of services. What equation represents Heather's gross profit?

ANSWER: Sales − Cost = Gross Profit or $30x − $18 = $162

B. How many manicures did Heather do?

STEP 1: Combine numbers and terms when possible.

$$\$30x − 18 = \$162$$

Note: There is nothing that can be combined because there is nothing that is alike.

STEP 2: Choose an algorithm to solve the equation. We will use the trial and error method.

STEP 3: Apply the algorithm to the equation, using 4 as a possible solution:

$$30x − 18 = 162$$
$$30(4) − 18 = 162$$
$$120 − 18 = 162$$

$102 \neq 162$ because 102 is smaller than 162; therefore, 4 is too small to be the solution. Try again to solve the problem, using a number that is larger than 4.

DID YOU KNOW? The trial and error method is a *guess and prove* method of solving equations.

STEP 4: Apply the algorithm to the equation using 8 as a possible solution:

$$30x − 18 = 162$$
$$30(8) − 18 = 162$$
$$240 − 18 = 162$$

$222 \neq 162$ because 222 is larger than 162; therefore, 8 is too large to be the solution.

STEP 5: Apply the algorithm to the equation, using 6 as a possible solution:

$$30x - 18 = 162$$
$$30(6) - 18 = 162$$
$$180 - 18 = 162$$

162 = 162 because the left and right side have the same value; therefore, 6 is the solution.

Heather did 6 manicures.

DID YOU KNOW? The addition method of solving an equation is used when the equation involves *addition* or *subtraction*.

QUESTION 2: **A.** Marco purchased 6 bottles of shampoo for $7 each. Marco wanted to make $10 on the sale of each bottle. What equation represents Marco's profit?

ANSWER: Sales − Cost = Gross Profit or $x - (6 \cdot 7) = 10 \cdot 6$

B. What were Marco's sales?

STEP 1: Combine numbers and terms when possible.

$$x - (6 \cdot 7) = 10 \cdot 6$$

Note: Consolidate by multiplying.

$$x - 42 = 60$$

STEP 2: Choose an algorithm to solve the equation. Let's use the addition method because the equation involves subtraction.

STEP 3: Apply the algorithm to the equation. **Note:** Eliminate by doing the opposite of the subtraction of 42 to both sides, or adding 42 to each side.

$$x - 42 = 60$$
$$x - 42 + 42 = 60 - 42 \text{ becomes } x - 0 = 102$$
$$x = 102$$

Let's prove our solution:

$$x - 42 = 60$$
$$102 - 42 = 60$$
$$60 = 60$$

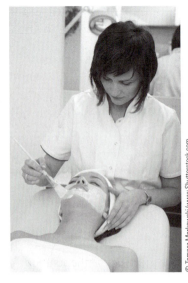

© Tomasz Markowski/www.Shutterstock.com

Marco's total sales were $102, because when we replace the variable with $102, both sides of the equation have the same value.

QUESTION 3: **A.** Amie charges $70 for a facial and made $490 in total sales. What equation represents Heather's total sales from facials?

Price × Quantity = Sales

ANSWER: $\$70x = \$490$

B. How many facials did Amie do?

ANSWER: **STEP 1:** Combine numbers and terms when possible.

$$\$70x = \$490$$

STEP 2: Choose an algorithm to solve the equation. In this case we will use the multiplication method because the equation involves multiplication.

STEP 3: Apply the algorithm to the equation. Note: eliminate by doing the opposite of the multiplication of 70 to both sides, or dividing each side by 70.

$$70x/70 = 490/70$$
$$x = 7$$

Let's prove our solution:

$$70x = 490$$
$$70(7) = 490$$
$$490 = 490$$

Amie did 7 facials, because when we replace the variable with 7, both sides of the equation have the same value.

DID YOU KNOW?   The multiplication method is used to solve an equation when the equation involves *multiplication* or *division.*

QUESTION 4:   **A.** Haley has an opportunity to sell hand lotion in her spa. She has 2 types to choose from. A case of the first type costs $52, and she thinks she can sell it for $8 a bottle. The second would sell for $6 a bottle and only cost her $32 for the case. If she decided to sell them both in the salon, how many of each type would she have to sell to earn the same amount of money? What equation will allow Haley to make the same amount of money under both scenarios?

ANSWER: First Scenario = Second Scenario
Sales − Cost = Sales − Cost
(Price × Quantity) − cost = (Price × Quantity) − cost
$8x − $52 = $6x − $32

B. How many bottles of hand lotion does Haley need to sell?

ANSWER: **STEP 1:** Combine numbers and terms when possible

$$\$8x - \$52 = \$6x - \$32$$

STEP 2: Choose an algorithm to solve the equation. Let's use the addition and multiplication methods because the problem involves *subtraction* and *multiplication.*

STEP 3: Apply the algorithm to the equation. Remember the addition method is always applied first. Add 52 to both sides.

$$8x - 52 + 52 = 6x - 32 + 52$$

becomes

$$8x = 6x + 20$$

STEP 4: Use the addition method again. Subtract 6x from both sides.

$$8x - 6x = 6x - 6x + 20$$

becomes

$$2x = 20$$

STEP 5: Use the multiplication method. Divide both sides by 2.

$2x/2 = 20/2$

$x = 10$

Let's prove our solution:

$8x - 52 = 6x - 32$

$8(10) - 52 = 6(10) - 32$

$80 - 52 = 60 - 32$

$28 = 28$

Haley needs to sell 10 bottles of hand lotion for both scenarios to have the same value.

6-1 LET ME TRY

1. Fefe charges $25 per manicure and paid a total of $10 for all her supplies. After subtracting the cost of supplies, she earned $65 on Tuesday.
   a. What equation represents Fefe's profit?

   b. Utilizing the trial and error method, how many manicures did Fefe sell?

2. Cheryl purchased 4 cans of finishing spray for $6 each. She wants to make a total profit of $36 from the sale of all 4 bottles.
   a. What equation represents Cheryl's gross profit?

   b. Utilizing the addition and multiplication methods, what was Cheryl's sales price per bottle?

3. Martine charges $60 for a full-head haircolor service and made a total of $540 from the sale of haircolor services for the week.
   a. What equation represents Martine's total haircolor sales?

   b. Utilizing the multiplication method, how many haircolor services did Martine perform?

4. Tishla is trying to determine how many regular and how many spa pedicures she has to sell to earn the same amount of money. Tishla charges $30 for a regular pedicure, and her total supply cost is $18; she charges $40 for a spa pedicure, and her total supply cost is $78.
   a. What equation represents the Tishla's situation?

   b. How many pedicures does Tishla need to sell of each type?

MEETING AND EXCEEDING PROFIT GOALS

Now that we understand how to use equations in business, it is time to move on to solving problems that may have one or *more* correct answers. Huh? More than one correct answer? You do it all the time. Here's an example:

April charges $35 for full set of gel nails. She bought a kit of gel product for $55 that says there is enough material in the kit to perform *at least* 30 full sets of gel nails. April knows that she must earn at least $155 for every $55 in product usage; so given these parameters, what is the least number of gel nail services, at $35 each, that she must provide?

How can there be more than one correct answer? There can be more than one correct answer because there will be an answer that indicates the *least* number of services April will need to provide to satisfy the profit margins she is working with, but then any number between that number and the number of services that can *potentially* be given if all of the product is used is also a correct answer.

So then, April must provide x number of services @ $35 each to meet her profits of $155 and cover her costs of $55.

The equation that symbolizes this is:

$155   the amount of money April must make for every $55 worth of product purchased

+ $55   the cost of the products needed to provide the services

= $35x$ the least number of services that need to be provided to meet the goals

$$\$155 + \$55 = 35x$$
$$\$210 = 35x$$
$$x = 210 \div 35$$
$$x = 6$$

So, April must perform *at least* 6 gel nail services @ $35 each to cover her profit and product cost requirements.

April can perform several more than 6 services, based on the amount of product she has to work with, but to make back the investment, she only needs to perform 6 services.

But that is still only one answer to the question, right? What if we replaced the x with 7, 8, or 9? Actually, we can replace x with any number between 6 (the least number of services April must perform) and 30 (the greatest number April can perform based on how much product she has to work with), and the answer will still be correct.

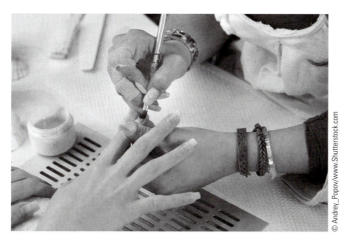
© Andrey_Popov/www.Shutterstock.com

After the least number of services (6) are performed, what kind of profit will be realized on any additional services performed with that product?

Yes! *Gross profit* will be realized on any additional services performed with that product. The answer is gross profit because we have not taken other types of expenses (such as overhead or salaries) into account.

QUESTION 1: Due to a pricing mistake, Patsy lost $3 on each bottle of nail polish she sold this week. Patsy's total losses were approximately $33. How many bottles of nail polish did Patsy sell?

ANSWER: **STEP 1:** Divide total loss by loss per bottle.

33	total loss on the nail polish for the week
÷ 3	loss per bottle
= 11	total number of bottles sold

QUESTION 2: Jessica charges $10 for a bottle of color-enhancing conditioner. Her total costs are $29, and she needs to earn a total profit of $71 or more from the sales of the color-enhancing conditioner. How many bottles of the conditioner does Jessica need to sell to earn a profit of at least $71?

ANSWER: **STEP 1:** Determine the amount that sales need to meet or exceed.

$29	Jessica's total costs for the conditioner
+ 71	the amount of profit Jessica needs to make on the sales of conditioner
= $100	total amount of money that sales need to equal or exceed

STEP 2: Divide total amount of sales by the sale price of each bottle.

$100	total amount of money that sales need to equal or exceed.
÷ 10	sales price of each bottle
10	number of bottles Jessica must sell to meet her goal

QUESTION 3: Marshall is competing in a haircutting competition in his salon. The person who first performs a total of $500 worth of haircuts in one week, will win. The prize is an educational haircutting class for free. If Marshall charges $32 for a shampoo, haircut, and styling, how many haircuts will he need to complete to win the contest?

ANSWER: **STEP 1:** Divide the total Marshall needs to achieve by the cost per haircut.

$500	the total sales of haircuts Marshall needs to achieve
÷ 32	the amount Marshall charges per haircut
15.625	the number of haircuts Marshall needs to accomplish to win

STEP 2: Round up.

15.625 = 16   total haircuts Marshall needs to accomplish to win

MAKING EXPENSE AND PROFIT PROJECTIONS

Previously we looked at equations that had only one unknown number, or where, if there was more than one unknown number, their values were equal. Now we will explore situations where there are two unknowns and they may not be equal.

Think that this is too farfetched a situation? Or that it cannot happen to you—after all, all you are doing is providing beauty and wellness services all day long. Try this on for size.

Let's say that you have $100 and have decided that you will invest that money in some new retail product to sell in the salon. You arrive at the distributor's store and realize that two items would sell well—cuticle oil and hand lotion. The hand lotion is $6 per bottle and the cuticle oil is $3 per bottle. How many of each can you purchase?

Aha! This is a situation where you have two unknown variables to try to figure out!

Because there can be several correct answers to this question, we will use the trial and error method to solve the problem. And because there are two *different* variables, we cannot use x for both, so we will use x for one and y for the other.

SHOW **ME** HOW

QUESTION 1: You have $100 and have decided that you will invest that money in some new retail product to sell in the salon. You arrive at the distributor's store and realize that two items would sell well—cuticle oil and hand lotion. The hand lotion is $6.00 per bottle and the cuticle oil is $3.00 per bottle. How many of each can you purchase?

ANSWER: **STEP 1:** Write an equation that represents the problem.

Cost of hand lotion + Cost of cuticle oil = $100

$6 × ?   + $3 × ?   = $100

$6x   + $3y   = $100

The equation is $6x + $3y = $100.

STEP 2: Determine how many bottles of each type of product you can purchase.

$6x + 3y = 100$	here's the original equation
$6(0) + 3y = 100$	this equation assumes that you will buy 0 bottles of hand lotion
$3y = 100$	this equation assumes that you will only buy cuticle oil
$3(33) = 99$	this equation tells you that you can buy 33 bottles of cuticle oil with $100

Therefore, you can buy zero bottles of hand lotion and 33 bottles of cuticle oil. Zero and 33 are possible solutions to this problem.

OR

$6x + 3y = 100$	here's the original equation
$6x + 3(0)y = 100$	this equation assumes that you will buy 0 bottles of cuticle oil
$6x = 100$	this equation assumes that you will only buy hand lotion
$6(16) = 96$	this equation tells you that you can buy 16 bottles of hand lotion with $100

Therefore, you can buy zero bottles of cuticle oil and 16 bottles of hand lotion. 0 and 16 are possible solutions to this problem.

STEP 3: Now you know that if you purchase less than 33 bottles of cuticle oil and less than 16 bottles of hand lotion, you can purchase both items. Remember, we are using the trial and error method—so let's see if we can purchase 8 bottles of hand lotion and 15 bottles of cuticle oil.

$$6x + 3y = 100$$
$$6(8) + 3(15) = 100$$
$$48 + 45 = 100$$
$$93 \neq 100$$

Although buying 8 bottles of hand lotion and 15 bottles of cuticle oil does not spend the entire budget of $100, it is a possible solution.

Or you can spend more of the budget by increasing the number of items you will buy. The difference between ($100 − $93 = $7) is enough to buy one more bottle of hand lotion or two more bottles of cuticle oil. So 9 and 15 could be the answer, or 8 and 17 could be the answer.

QUESTION 2: Joanna charges $40 for a full set of sculptured nails and $20 for a fill-in. Joanna earned a total sales of $320 today. How many of each service could Joanna have done today?

ANSWER: **STEP 1:** Write an equation that represents the problem.

$$\text{Full set} + \text{Fill ins} = \$320$$
$$\$40 \times ? + \$20 \times ? = \$320$$
$$\$40x + \$20y = \$320$$

STEP 2: Now determine how many of each service Joanna would have to perform to make $320.

$40x + 20y = 320$	the original equation
$40x + 20(0) = 320$	this equation assumes that joanna performed no fill-in services
$40x = 320$	this equation assumes that joanna only performed full-set services
$320 \div 40 = 8$	the total number of full sets Joanna could have performed is 8

8 and 0 are possible solutions to this problem.

OR

$40x + 20y = 320$	the original equation
$40(0) + 20x = 320$	this equation assumes that Joanna performed no full-set services
$20x = 320$	this equation assumes that Joanna only performed fill-in services
$320 \div 20 = 16$	the total number of fill-in services Joanna could have performed is 16

0 and 16 are possible solutions to this problem.

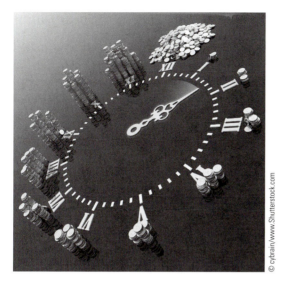

© cybrain/www.Shutterstock.com

STEP 3: Now you know that if Joanna performs less than 8 full sets and 16 fill-ins, she likely performed both services—so let's see how many fill-ins Joanna performed if she performed 5 full sets in a day.

$40x + 20y = 320$	the original equation
$40(5) + 20y = 320$	this equation assumes that Joanna performed 5 full-set services
$200 + 20y = 320$	total value of 5 full sets plus y equals 320
$20y = 320 - 200$	this equation assumes that 320 minus the sales of 5 full sets equals $20y$
$20y = 120$	in this equation $20y$ equals 120
$y = 120 \div 20$	in this equation y equals 120 divided by 20
$y = 6$	number of fill-ins Joanna performed if she performed 5 full sets

The answer to this scenario is 5, 6. If Joanna performs 5 full sets, she will need to perform 6 fill-ins to make $320 in a day.

6-2 LET ME TRY

Here's an equation for you to solve on your own.

Lonnie has $40 to purchase two different types of shampoo. Shampoo "x" costs $5 per bottle and shampoo "y" costs $8 per bottle. How many bottles of each type of shampoo can Lonnie purchase?

a. Write an equation that represents the problem.

b. How many bottles of each type of shampoo can Lonnie purchase? Give at least 3 solutions.

DETERMINING MINIMUM EXPECTATIONS

Remember that in the last chapter we discussed inequalities. Inequalities are mathematical statements that say two things have different values. Inequalities are comparison symbols that allow for an infinite amount of solutions. Symbols that denote inequalities are:

$\leq$ This symbol means that the numbers to the left of the symbol are *less than* or *equal to* the numbers on the right of the symbol.

≥ This symbol means that the numbers to the left of the symbol are *greater than* or *equal to* the numbers on the right of the symbol.

< This symbol means that the numbers to the left of the symbol are *less than* the numbers on the right of the symbol.

> This symbol means that the numbers to the left of the symbol are *greater than* the numbers on the right of the symbol.

You will also find that sometimes, when dealing with inequalities, we have to deal with a boundary. A **boundary** is a restriction on the solution that does not allow the solution to extend or go beyond a certain point called the *upper* or *lower limits* of the solution. The boundary may be found by substituting the inequality sign for an equal sign and then solving the problem. The boundary is where the solution must stop or begin.

What kind of a beauty-related situation could occur that could possibly leave you dealing with boundaries? And how would you resolve it?

SHOW ME HOW

QUESTION 1: Gina is on her way to purchase supplies and realizes that she cannot spend any more than $140, because that is what is in her checking account right now. She intends to purchase permanent waving solution at $12 per box and gloves at $10 per box. How many supplies can Gina purchase without going over her budget?

ANSWER: **STEP 1:** Write an inequality to represent the problem.

$12x + $10y < $140

STEP 2: Determine how many boxes of perm solution Gina can buy without exceeding her budget (boundary).

$12x + 10y < 140$	the original equation
$12x + 10(0) < 140$	this equation assumes that Gina does not buy gloves
$12x < 140$	this equation assumes that Gina only buys perm solution
$x = 140 \div 12$	divide the budget by the price of the perm solution
$x = 11.66$	the number of boxes of perm solution that can be purchased with $140
$x = 11$	because .66 of a box of perm solution cannot be purchased and rounding up would exceed the budget (boundary), we round down
$12(11) + 10(0) < 140$	this equation indicates that one solution to the equation is 11 and 0

STEP 3: Determine how many boxes of gloves Gina can buy without exceeding her budget (boundary).

$12x + 10y < 140$	the original equation
$12(0) + 10y < 140$	this equation assumes that Gina does not buy perm solution
$10y < 140$	this equation assumes that Gina only buys gloves
$y = 140 \div 10$	divide the budget by the price of the gloves
$y = 14$	the number of boxes of gloves that can be purchased with $140
$x = 13$	because the original equation indicates that Gina needs to spend less than $140, the correct solution is 13
$12(0) + 10(13) < 140$	this equation indicates that one solution to the equation is 0 and 13

STEP 4: Now we know that Gina can purchase as many as 11 boxes of perm solution or 13 boxes of gloves. If Gina wants to buy both, we know that she needs to purchase less than 11 boxes of perm solution and 13 boxes of gloves. Let's see if we can meet the $140 budget if Gina purchases 10 boxes of perm solution and 3 boxes of gloves.

$12x + 10y < 140$	the original equation
$12(10) + 10(3) < 140$	this equation assumes Gina purchases 10 boxes of perm solution and 3 boxes of gloves
$120 + 30 < 140$	totals of all purchases
$150 < 140$	this equation shows that if Gina makes the purchase, she will have exceeded the budget (boundary)

STEP 5: Reduce the number of purchases and try the equation again.

$12x + 10y < 140$	the original equation
$12(9) + 10(3) < 140$	this equation assumes that Gina purchases 9 boxes of perm solution and 3 boxes of gloves
$108 + 30 < 140$	totals of all purchases
$138 < 140$	this equation shows that if Gina makes the purchase, she will have remained under the budget (boundary)

One solution to this problem is 9 and 3.

QUESTION 2: Olivia charges an average of $50 per hour for her services, overhead cost is $20 per hour, and the total cost of her supplies is $150 per week. Olivia wants to know the minimum number of hours she needs to work in order for her total sales to be more than her total costs.

ANSWER: **STEP 1:** Write an inequality to represent the problem.

$$\$50y > \$20x + \$150$$

STEP 2: Assume that 6 hours are worked and determine the minimum number of hours Olivia needs to work to achieve her goal.

$\$50y > \$20x + \$150$	the original equation
$50(6) > \$20(6) + \$150$	the equation assumes that 6 hours are worked. And although y is 6 (number of hours worked), y is also 6 because the costs incurred are calculated per hour worked, and 6 is the total number of hours
$300 > 120 + 150$	calculations on both sides of the symbol
$300 > 270$	a correct assumption

Olivia needs to work a minimum of 6 hours for her sales to exceed her costs.

1. What is an equation and how is it used in calculating profits?

2. Define an algorithm and name the three types used in solving equations.

3. What is the trial and error method of solving an equation?

4. Define the addition method of solving an equation and explain when it is used.

5. Define the multiplication method of solving an equation and explain when it is used.

Budgeting, Planning, and Reporting

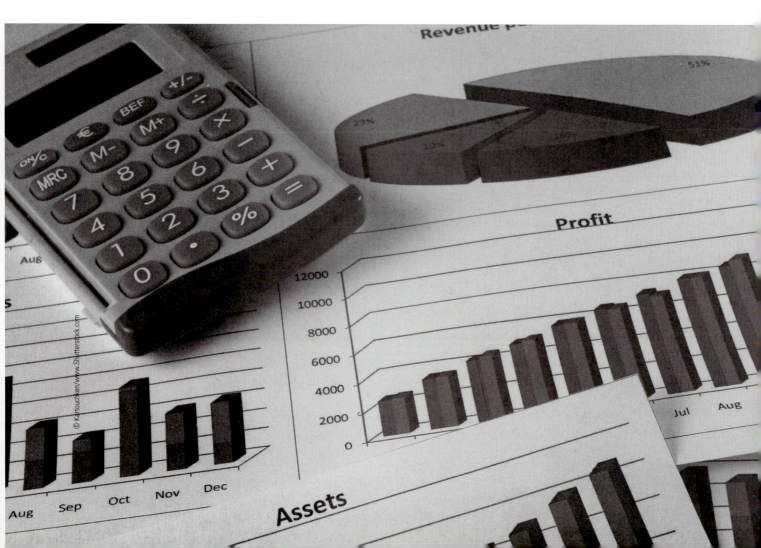

- Graphs
- Business Reporting

- Sales Forecasting

LEARNING OBJECTIVES

After completing this chapter, you will be able to:

1. Understand the use of graphs used in business reporting and what they can illustrate.

2. Explain the use of correlations in business reporting.

3. Recognize and read an income statement and balance sheet.

4. Know the difference between revenues and expenses.

5. Perform the necessary calculations to determine percentage of revenue for each service offered in a salon or spa.

6. Compare and contrast figures from current and past financial statements.

7. Explain the difference between variable and fixed costs.

8. Define the break-even point of a business.

KEY TERMS

- assets
- balance sheet
- bar graph
- break-even point
- correlation
- creditors

- expense
- fixed costs
- graph
- income statement
- liabilities
- line graph

- net profit
- owner's equity
- pie graph
- ratio
- revenue
- variable costs

N THE BEAUTY AND WELLNESS FIELDS, CLIENTS OFTEN BRING IN PHOTOS and ask to have a desired hairstyle, haircolor, or makeup style emulated. The familiar saying "A picture is worth a thousand words" certainly holds true in these instances because the photo explains—far better than the client alone probably could—the look she is trying to achieve. Photos are extremely helpful to beauty and wellness professionals because they help us understand a certain idea or concept through the use of a very vivid and precise visual aid.

In mathematics and business, numbers are used to create pictures, and these too can be very helpful for seeing particular patterns, trends, or gaps in the overall financial health and well-being a of a business.

GRAPHS

A **graph** is a mathematical picture that expresses or defines a solution to a problem. Like most pictures, a graph can express a solution in a way that is easy to understand. A graph is a picture that allows us to compare and establish patterns regarding numbers and outcomes. This is very important, because it allows us to see what has occurred over an extended period of time and allows us to use that past history to make predictions about what is likely to happen in the future. These pictures also give us clues as to where opportunities may lie for increasing sales, services, and promotions, as well as helping us to realize places where we can save time, energy, and money.

A graph allows us to contrast distinct differences to changing situations in a manner that numbers and words never could. Besides being easy to understand, graphs also provide a high level of professionalism in the presentation of a solution or outcome. Graphs allow the reader to know that the presenter of the information has made an effort to examine the relationships among various concepts and how the concepts might affect future outcomes.

Let's take a look at several types of graphs, such as pie graphs, bar graphs, and line graphs, and discover how these graphs can be used in a day spa or wellness setting.

Characteristics of Graphs

There are various ways that graphs can present a mathematical picture that expresses or defines a solution to a problem. Graphs should always be read from left to right, just like a textbook. All graphs are two-dimensional in that they have to be viewed from two directions. Most of the time, a graph requires the reader to view the graph vertically and horizontally at the same time. The two-dimensional aspect of a graph shows the reader that there is a **correlation**, or a relationship between two things—in this case the numbers represented both vertically and the numbers represented horizontally on the graph. The correlation is a pattern that allows the reader to observe the past and make predictions about the future based upon the past.

Many things share a relationship with other things. An example is the time spent studying compared to the grade earned in a class. The more a student studies, the greater his or her chances are of passing a class. Based on this information, if a student never studied, we could safely deduce that the student would have a more difficult time passing a class. On the other hand, if a student studied a lot, we could safely deduce that the student would have a better chance of passing a class.

Graphs, such a pie graphs, bar graphs, and line graphs, are used to help us see complex patterns that are not easy to recognize otherwise. A **pie graph**, also known as *pie chart*, is a circular graph that uses pie shapes to compare and contrast numerical values. The following is an example of a pie chart.

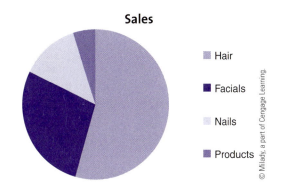

A **bar graph** (see below) is a graph that uses rectangular shapes to compare and contrast numerical values.

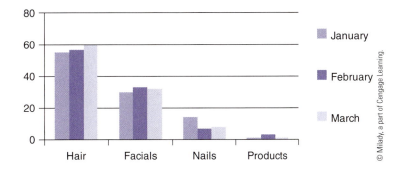

A **line graph** is a graph that uses straight lines to compare and contrast numerical values. Line graphs, as shown below, can only be used to examine relationships between data that have a direct or inverse relationship.

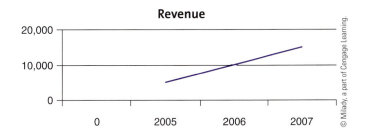

Many graphs use or define a ratio. A **ratio** is a process that compares two quantities by the basic operation of division. For example, if we were trying to determine the ratio of revenue from facials to the revenue of a spa where the total revenue is $4,000 and the revenue from facials is $1,200, the mathematical equation would look like this:

$$\frac{Facials}{Total\ Revenue} = \frac{1,200}{4,000} = \frac{1,200 \div 400}{4,000 \div 400} = \frac{3}{10} = .30 = 30\%$$

BUSINESS REPORTING

Many beauty and wellness professionals prefer to perform services and interact with clients while dismissing thoughts about how well their business is doing. It is irresponsible to make excuses like "I'm not good with numbers" or "I just want to formulate haircolor and let someone else worry about the numbers." Nowadays there are excellent computerized programs that make dealing with business revenues and expenses easier to manage, and with the touch of a button, business reports can be generated that explain the entire situation. Although many calculators, software programs, and even accountants and accounting firms that you will work with in your career will do a lot of the work for you in generating these reports, it is important for you to know what the numbers represent and how the calculations were arrived at.

Unfortunately, no report can be very helpful if it is not read or understood. Let's take a look at some of the common types of reports you need to be familiar with and an explanation of what the reports are showing you.

An **income statement** is a financial report that compares the company's income, expense, and net profit. The following is an example of an income statement.

Jonathon's Day Spa Income Statement Year Ending December 31, ####	
Revenue:	
Body Treatments	$ 67,600
Facials	$ 27,850
Massage	$ 24,450
Retail Sales	$ 5,100
Total Revenue	$125,000
Less: Cost of Products Sold	$ 3,570
Gross Profit	$ 121,430
Expenses:	
Rent	$ 24,000
Utilities	$ 1,800
Taxes & Licenses	$ 2,100
Depreciation	$ 1,600
Supplies (service related)	$ 15,300
Travel	$ 1,600
Office Supplies	$ 1,350
Telephone	$ 960
Advertising	$ 4,250
Labor	$ 18,720
Total Expenses	$ 71,680
NET PROFIT	$ 49,750

A **balance sheet** is a financial report that compares a company's assets, liabilities, and equity (see below).

Jonathon's Day Spa Income Statement Year Ending December 31, ####	
Assets:	
Cash	$ 18,700
Supplies (product)	$ 7,400
Office Supplies	$ 650
Equipment	$16,000
Total Assets	$ 42,750
Liabilities:	
Accounts Payable (suppliers)	$ 1,275
Notes Payables (business loan)	$15,000
Total Liabilities	$ 16,275
Owner's Equity:	
Paid in Capital (owner's investment)	$ 18,675
Retained Profit (less withdrawals)	$ 7,800
Total Equity	$ 26,475
Total Liabilities and Owner's Equity:	$ 42,750

On these reports you will see numbers representing:

- **Revenue**, which is the income that a company generates through sales from services and products.
- **Expense**, which is the cost or bills that a company pays, such as rent, utilities, supplies, telephone, advertising, and so on.
- **Net profit**, which is the difference between the revenue and expenses.
- **Assets**, which are items that a company owns that can generate money or be converted into money—these can include equipment, supplies, money, land, and buildings.
- **Liabilities**, also known as *debt*; this is the amount of money that the company owes for such things as mortgage notes, car loans, revolving lines of credit, notes payable, and accounts payable.
- **Creditors** are the people to whom the money is owed, and creditors have rights to the assets of a company if the company cannot pay their debts.
- **Owner's equity** is the difference between the assets and liabilities. The owner has rights to the assets after the creditors have been paid.

Business Reporting Using Graphs

As we've already discussed, graphs are great ways to show, in picture form, the numbers that represent a business's financial health, growth, or decline. At some point in your career, you may need to borrow money for an expansion, to open a second location, or to invest in equipment that you feel will lead to greater sales, and you may need to prove to a banker or investor that the monies are justified. Graphing your past sales, growth, and revenues is an excellent way of making a financial point.

Let's take a look at a good example of this. Several years ago, a local bank gave Jonathon his first business loan to open his day spa. Now Jonathon wants to apply for another loan to expand and improve his day spa. Although the day spa seems to be busy and has a great reputation, the bank wants to see some reporting that will justify the loan, such as graphs that show how Jonathon's business has progressed over the years.

EXAMPLE 1

Jonathon decides to create a pie graph to compare and contrast various service revenue to total revenue from his day spa. The information from Jonathon's income statement will be used to complete the graph. All numbers will be rounded to the nearest hundredth of a decimal.

Sources	Ratios	Decimal Form	Percentage
Body Treatments	67,600/125,000	.5408	54%
Facials	27,850/125,000	.2228	22%
Massage	24,450/125,000	.1956	20%
Retail sales	5,100/125,000	.0408	4%
Total	25,000/125,000	1.0000	100%

Based on these numbers from the income statement, here is what the pie chart looks like:

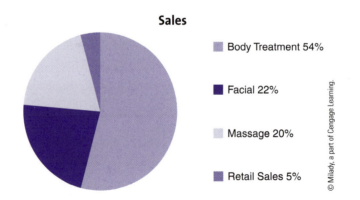

Sales

- Body Treatment 54%
- Facial 22%
- Massage 20%
- Retail Sales 5%

EXAMPLE 2

Jonathon decides to create a pie graph to compare and contrast liabilities to total assets and owner's equity to total assets. The information from his balance sheet will be used to complete the graph. All numbers will be rounded to the nearest hundredth of a decimal.

Item	Ratios	Decimal Form	Percent Form
Liabilities	16,275/42,750	.3807	38%
Owner's Equity	26,475/42,750	.6193	62%
Assets	42,750/42,750	1.0000	100%

Based on these numbers from the balance sheet, here is what the pie chart looks like:

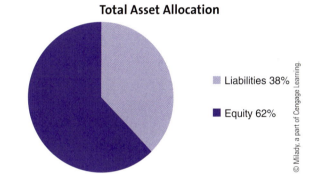

Total Asset Allocation

Liabilities 38%

Equity 62%

EXAMPLE 3

Jonathon decides to create a bar graph to compare and contrast revenue. The information from his income statement will be used to complete the graph.

Sources	Amount
Body Treatments	$ 67,600
Facials	$ 27,850
Massage	$ 24,450
Retail Sales	$ 5,100
Total	$125,000

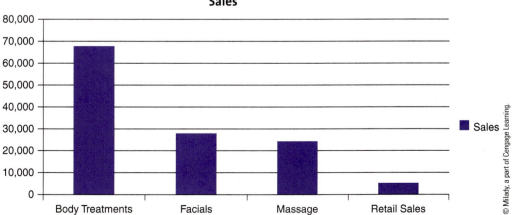

Sales

EXAMPLE 4

Jonathon decides to create a bar graph to compare and contrast his liabilities, equity, and assets. The information from Jonathon's balance sheet will be used to complete the graph.

Item	Amount
Assets	$42,750
Liabilities	$16,275
Equity	$25,475

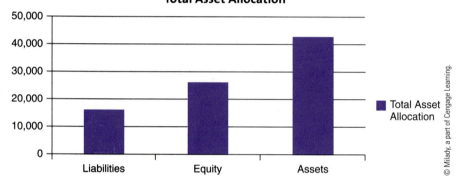

EXAMPLE 5

Jonathon decides to create a line graph to compare and contrast total revenue from current and prior years. The information below will be used to create a line graph.

Total Revenue	
2008	$118,000
2009	$163,000
2010	$ 89,000
2011	$111,000
2012	$125,000

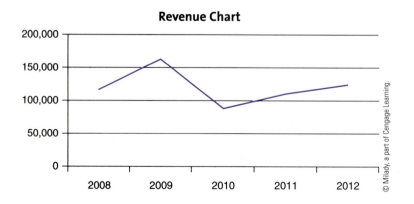

1. Jonathon decides to create a pie graph to compare and contrast expenses. Please use the information from his income statement to complete the table below. All decimals will be rounded to the nearest hundredth of a decimal. The information is in the figure on page 104.

Source of Expenses	Identify the Ratios	Convert to a Decimal	Convert to a Percent
1.			
2.			
3.			
4.			
5.			
6.			
7.			
8.			
9.			
10.			
Expenses $71,680	$71,680/$71,680	1.00	100%

Now that you have completed filling in the information in the table above, which of the following graphs represents the expenses of Jonathon's Day Spa: Graph A or Graph B?

Graph A

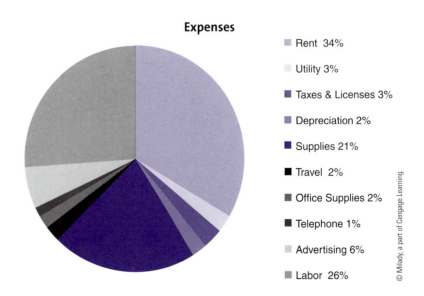

Expenses

- Rent 34%
- Utility 3%
- Taxes & Licenses 3%
- Depreciation 2%
- Supplies 21%
- Travel 2%
- Office Supplies 2%
- Telephone 1%
- Advertising 6%
- Labor 26%

Graph B

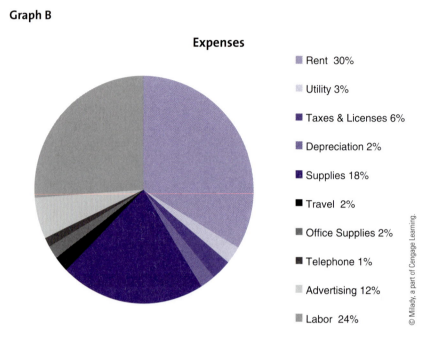

Expenses

- Rent 30%
- Utility 3%
- Taxes & Licenses 6%
- Depreciation 2%
- Supplies 18%
- Travel 2%
- Office Supplies 2%
- Telephone 1%
- Advertising 12%
- Labor 24%

© Milady, a part of Cengage Learning.

Please explain your answer.

_____

_____

_____

_____

2. Jonathon decides to create a bar graph to compare and contrast expenses. Please use the information from his income statement to complete the problem. The information is in the figure on page 104.

	Source	Amounts
1.		
2.		
3.		
4.		
5.		
6.		
7.		
8.		
9.		
10.		
Total Expenses		$71,680

© Milady, a part of Cengage Learning.

Which bar graph below represents the expenses of Jonathon's Day Spa: Graph A or Graph B?

Graph A

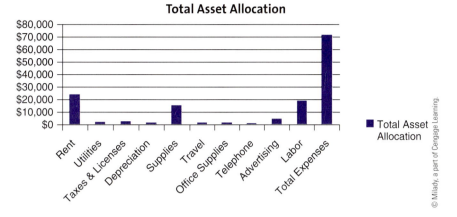

Graph B

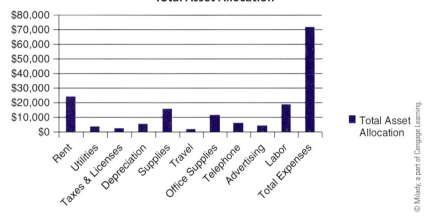

Please explain your answer.

_____

_____

_____

_____

3. Jonathon decides to create a line graph to compare and contrast net profit from the current and prior years. Please use the information below to create the line graph.

Net Profit	
2012	$49,750
2011	$61,300
2010	$40,675
2009	$46,232
2008	$43,128

Create a graph that will represent Jonathon's net profit.

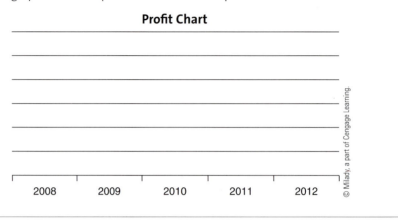

Profit Chart

2008   2009   2010   2011   2012

© Milady, a part of Cengage Learning.

SALES FORECASTING

In order to keep your business fresh and healthy, it is useful to take a look at where your total sales have been in the past and to use that information to plan and set goals for the future. All businesses—whether salons, spas, fast-food franchises, or car dealerships—use sales forecasting as a means of setting goals for the coming year. The goal is not a number someone picked out of thin air; however, it should be a number that is determined by looking at where the business has been and how it has performed. Once the forecasts are determined, the information can be graphed for a quick and easy way to review it.

There are a few accounting terms to be aware of as we perform these calculations. They are:

- **Variable costs** are costs that are directly linked to the ability to service a client and will increase or decrease as the number of clients increases or decreases.

- **Fixed costs** are costs or expenses that never or rarely change. Fixed cost may include: rent, utilities, licenses, fees, tax, telephone, and depreciation.

- **Break-even point** is an equation that defines a point where the revenue and cost are the same, or even.

Let's try doing some sales forecasting now, using Jonathon's Day Spa sales numbers for the past few years.

SHOW ME HOW

QUESTION 1: Jonathon decides to create a graph to get a better understanding of his ability to generate revenue. Jonathon's revenue for 2011 consisted of: Body Treatments of $60,000; Facials of $35,000; Massage of $30,000; and Retail Sales of $20,015. Jonathon's appointment book indicates that his day spa serviced 2,231 clients in 2011. Based on these findings, what is a reasonable forecast for Jonathon's Day Spa's revenue for 2012?

ANSWER: **STEP 1:** Create an equation to represent Jonathon's ability to generate revenue in 2012 based upon his 2011 earnings.

Revenue = Average Price × No. of Clients

STEP 2: Determine the average price each client paid by adding together all of the revenues for 2011 and dividing it by the number of clients serviced.

$\quad$ $60,000 $\quad$ body treatments
+ $ 35,000 $\quad$ facials
+ $ 30,000 $\quad$ massage
+ $ 20,015 $\quad$ retail sales
$\quad$ $145,015 $\quad$ total revenue in 2011
$\quad$ $145,015 $\quad$ total revenue in 2011
$\quad$ ÷ 2,231 $\quad$ number of clients serviced in 2011
$\quad\quad$ $65 $\quad$ average price each client paid for services, including retail sales

STEP 3: Create a table using 2 variables: x = number of clients serviced and y = revenue for that service, based on the average client sale in 2011 ($65).

$\quad\quad x \quad\quad\quad y$

Clients/Revenues

1,000/$65,000	This ratio assumes that if 1,000 clients pay $65 each, revenue will equal $65,000.
1,500/$97,500	This ratio assumes that if 1,500 clients pay $65 each, revenue will equal $97,500.
2,000/$130,000	This ratio assumes that if 2,000 clients pay $65 each, revenue will equal $130,000.
2,500/$162,500	This ratio assumes that if 2,500 clients pay $65 each, revenue will equal $162,500.
3,000/$195,000	This ratio assumes that if 3,000 clients pay $65 each, revenue will equal $195,000.
3,500/$227,500	This ratio assumes that if 3,500 clients pay $65 each, revenue will equal $227,500.

STEP 4: Create a linear graph.

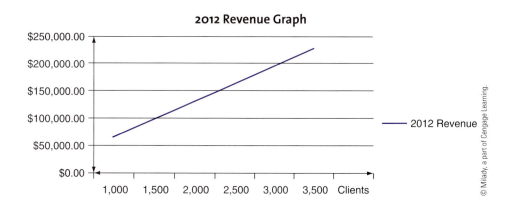

Based on this graph, Jonathon can see that the more clients his spa services, the greater his revenues will be. He can do additional calculations to determine how many more clients he serviced in 2011 than in 2010 and use that number (in percentage form) to estimate how many more clients he can service in 2012 than in 2011, thus forecasting his sales increase.

QUESTION 2: Jonathon decides to create a graph to get a better understanding of his total cost in 2012 based upon his 2011 total revenue. Jonathon's fixed cost for the prior year, 2011, consisted of: Rent $24,000; Utilities $1,800; Taxes/Licenses $2,100; Depreciation $1,600; Telephone $960; and Advertising $4,250. Jonathon's variable cost for the prior year, 2008, consists of: Products/Supplies $15,626; Office Supplies $1,350; and Labor $18,720. Jonathon's appointment book indicates that his day spa serviced 2,231 clients in 2011. What could Jonathon's total costs for 2012 be?

ANSWER: **STEP 1:** Create an equation to represent Jonathon's total cost for 2012 based upon his 2011 cost.

Total Cost = (Average Variable Cost ÷ No. of Clients) + Fixed Cost

STEP 2: Add up both the variable costs and the fixed costs.

Variable Costs

$ 18,720	labor
+$ 15,626	supplies
+$ 1,350	office supplies
$35,696	total variable costs for 2011

Fixed Costs

$24,000	rent
+ $ 1,800	utilities
+ $ 2,100	taxes/licenses
+ $ 1,600	depreciation
+ $ 960	telephone
+ $ 4,250	advertising
$34,710	total fixed costs for 2011

STEP 3: Fill in the equation with the correct numbers.

Total Cost = (Average Variable Cost ÷ No. of Clients) + Fixed Cost
Total Cost = ($35,696 ÷ 2232) + $34,710
Total Cost = $16 × (No. of Clients) + $34,710

STEP 4: Create a table.

x y

Clients/Total Cost

0/$34,710	Even if there are 0 clients incurring variable costs, the business still has its fixed costs to pay.
500/$42,710	If the spa services 500 clients @ $16 each for variable costs plus the fixed costs, the total equals $42,710.
1,000/$50,710	If the spa services 1,000 clients @ $16 each for variable costs plus the fixed costs, the total equals $50,710.
1,500/$58,710	If the spa services 1,500 clients @ $16 each for variable costs plus the fixed costs, the total equals $58,710.
2,000/$66,710	If the spa services 2,000 clients @ $16 each for variable costs plus the fixed costs, the total equals $66,710.
2,500/$74,710	If the spa services 2,500 clients @ $16 each for variable costs plus the fixed costs, the total equals $74,710.

| 3,000/$82,710 | If the spa services 3,000 clients @ $16 each for variable costs plus the fixed costs, the total equals $82,710. |
| 3,500/$90,710 | If the spa services 3,500 clients @ $16 each for variable costs plus the fixed costs, the total equals $90,710. |

STEP 5: Create a line graph with these numbers.

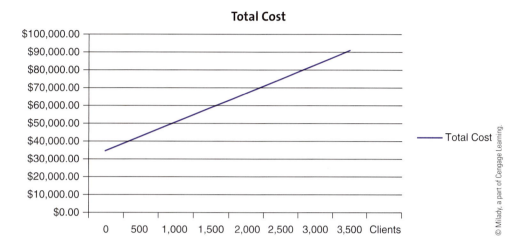

QUESTION 3: Jonathon needs to know what his break-even point for 2012 will be. He will use the information arrived at in questions 1 and 2 to get his answer.

ANSWER: **STEP 1:** Find the revenue equation.

Revenue = Price × Client

Revenue = $65 × (No. of clients serviced)

$\quad x \qquad y$

Clients/Revenues

1,000/$65,000	This ratio assumes that if 1,000 clients pay $65 each, revenue will equal $65,000.
1,500/$97,500	This ratio assumes that if 1,500 clients pay $65 each, revenue will equal $97,500.
2,000/$130,000	This ratio assumes that if 2,000 clients pay $65 each, revenue will equal $130,000.
2,500/$162,500	This ratio assumes that if 2,500 clients pay $65 each, revenue will equal $162,500.
3,000/$195,000	This ratio assumes that if 3,000 clients pay $65 each, revenue will equal $195,000.
3,500/$227,500	This ratio assumes that if 3,500 clients pay $65 each, revenue will equal $227,500.

STEP 2: Find the cost equation.

Total Cost = (Average Variable Cost ÷ No. of Clients) + Fixed Cost

Total Cost = ($35,696 ÷ 2232) + $34,710

Total Cost = $16 × (No. of Clients) + $34,710

x   *y*

Clients/Total Cost

0/$34,710	Even if there are 0 clients incurring variable costs, the business still has its fixed costs to pay.
500/$42,710	If the spa services 500 clients @ $16 each for variable costs plus the fixed costs, the total equals $42,710.
1,000/$50,710	If the spa services 1,000 clients @ $16 each for variable costs plus the fixed costs, the total equals $50,710.
1,500/$58,710	If the spa services 1,500 clients @ $16 each for variable costs plus the fixed costs, the total equals $58,710.
2,000/$66,710	If the spa services 2,000 clients @ $16 each for variable costs plus the fixed costs, the total equals $66,710.
2,500/$74,710	If the spa services 2,500 clients @ $16 each for variable costs plus the fixed costs, the total equals $74,710.
3,000/$82,710	If the spa services 3,000 clients @ $16 each for variable costs plus the fixed costs, the total equals $82,710.
3,500/$90,710	If the spa services 3,500 clients @ $16 each for variable costs plus the fixed costs, the total equals $90,710.

STEP 3: Combine the equations to find the break-even point. The break-even point is when the revenue equals the costs.

Revenue = Cost

$65 \times$ (No. of Clients) = $16x$ (No. of Clients) + 34,710

$65x - 16x = 16x - 16x + 34{,}710$ Simplify by combining like terms and doing the same function to both sides of the equation.

$49x = 34{,}710$

$x = 34{,}710 \div 49$

$x = 708.367$

Therefore, if Jonathon services 708 to 709 clients in a year, he will break even. His revenue and expenses will be the same.

STEP 4: Create a graph of each equation to show the break-even point.

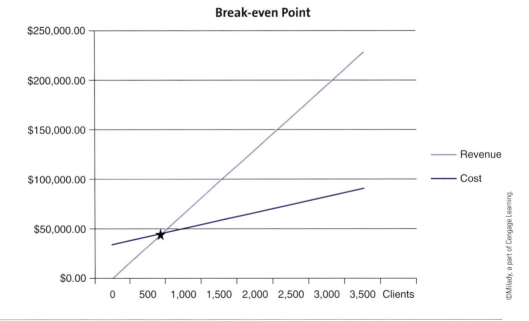

Break-even Point

1. Create a graph to get a better understanding of Jonathon's ability to generate revenue in 2011 based upon his 2010 total revenue. Jonathon's 2010 revenue consisted of: Body Treatments of $55,000; Facials of $36,000; Massage of $27,000; and Retail Sales of $22,000. Jonathon's appointment book indicates that his day spa serviced 2,000 clients in 2010.

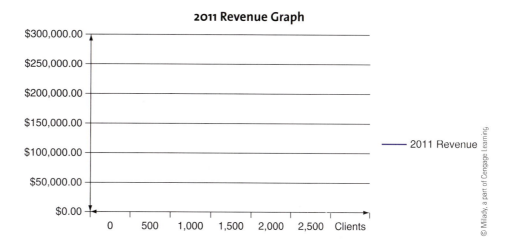

2. Create a graph to get a better understanding of Jonathon's total cost in 2011 based upon his total cost in 2010. Jonathon's fixed costs for the prior year, 2010, consisted of: Rent of $22,000; Utilities of $1,900; Taxes/Licenses of $2,000; Depreciation of $1,600; Telephone of $1,000; and Advertising of $3,900. Jonathon's variable cost for the prior year, 2010, consisted of: Products/Supplies $20,400; Office Supplies $1,600; and Labor $18,000. Jonathon's appointment book indicates that his day spa serviced 2,000 clients in 2010.

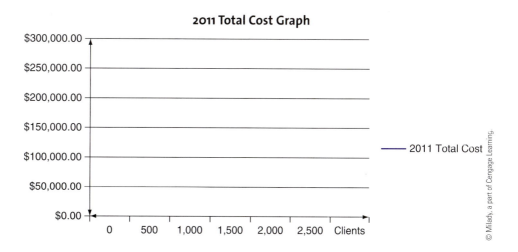

3. Use the information from question 1 and question 2 to find Jonathon's break-even point for 2011.

Break-even Point

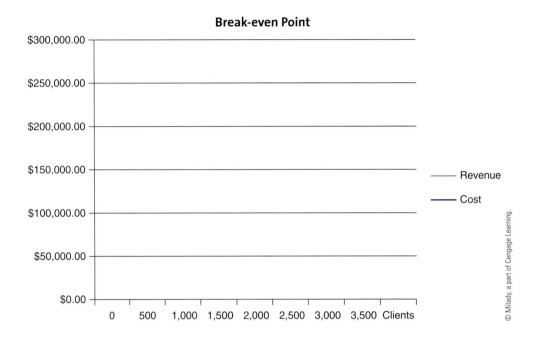

4. Take a look at the following graph. What information does it indicate to you?

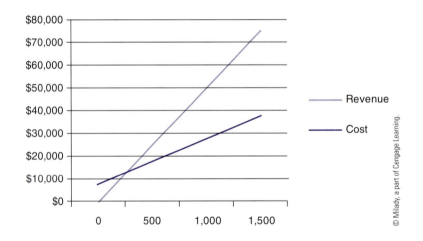

5. Take a look at the following graph. What information does it indicate to you?

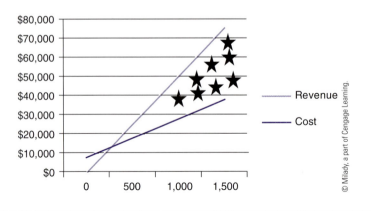

1. How are graphs used in business reporting, and what do they allow you to see?

2. Define correlations. Why are they important in business reporting?

3. What information is found on an income statement? What information is found on a balance sheet?

4. What is the difference between revenue and expense?

5. Describe how to determine percentage of revenue for each service offered in a salon or spa.

6. Describe the type of graph that allows you to compare and contrast figures from current and past financial statements.

7. Explain the difference between variable and fixed costs, and give examples of each.

8. What is a business's break-even point?

Inventory Control Using the Metric System

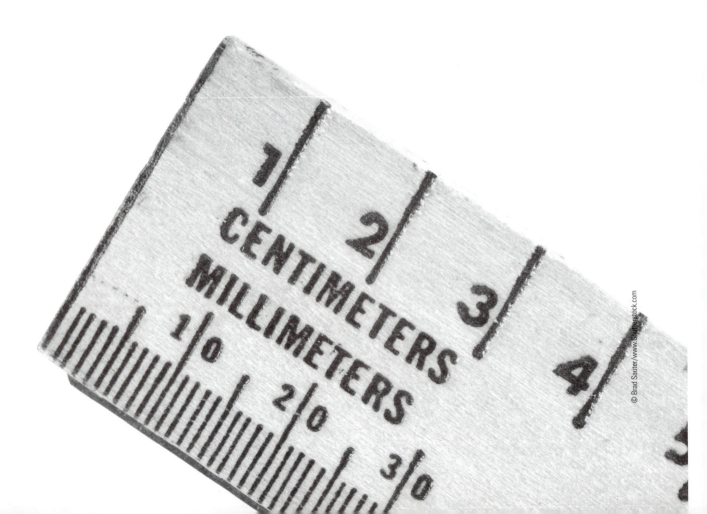

- Types of Measurement
- Converting Measurements

LEARNING OBJECTIVES

After completing this chapter, you will be able to:

1. Identify the various types of measurement systems.

2. Recognize how each measurement system measures distance, mass, and volume.

3. Name the steps involved in converting measurement from one system to the other.

KEY TERMS

- conversion rate
- converting multiple rates
- cross multiplication
- English measurement
- metric measurement
- rate
- unit measurement

AVE YOU EVER NOTICED THAT YOUR BACKBAR AND RETAIL PRODUCTS have a variety of measurements on their labels? In the beauty and wellness industry you will find products sold in gallons, liters, milliliters, grams, pounds, pints, or quarts. It can be very frustrating trying to compare costs and volume of products when they use different measuring systems.

In this chapter, we are going to take a look at the various types of measurement systems and learn how to convert one type of measurement to another, so evaluating the product or its price is easier. This will be an invaluable skill in further controlling inventory and managing your product spending.

TYPES OF MEASUREMENT

Unit measurement is a way of defining an item in numerical terms that allows the quantity of the item to be compared to the quantity of another item. In measurement systems, distance is measured in meters, yards, miles, inches, and feet. Solids or weight are measured in grams and pounds, and volume or liquid is measured in liters, gallons, pints, or quarts.

There are two types of unit measurement that are used globally; they are *English measurement* and *metric measurement*. Metric measurement is also known as the metric system.

English measurement is a system of measurements that measures solids, liquids, and distance with different measurement units depending on the quantity and type of item.

In terms of distance, English measurement states that 12 inches equal 1 foot; 3 feet equal 1 yard; and 1760 yards equal 1 mile. When measuring mass or weight, English measurement states that 16 ounces (abbreviated oz) equal 1 pound, and 2,000 pounds equal 1 ton. In the case of volume or measuring liquid, 8 ounces equal 1 cup; 2 cups equal 1 pint; 2 pints equal 1 quart; and 4 quarts equal 1 gallon.

Metric measurement, also known as *the metric system*, is a system of measurement that measure solids, liquids, and distance with three basic units. The three basic units are: *grams*, *liters*, and *meters*. The three basic units can be increased or decreased with pre-fixes. The prefixes used in metric measurement are:

- Kilo, meaning one thousand (1000)
- Hecto, meaning one hundred (100)
- Deca, meaning ten (10)
- Deci, meaning tenth (.1)
- Centi, meaning hundredth (.01)
- Milli, meaning thousandth (.001)

When measuring distance:

- 1 kilometer equals 1,000 meters
- 1 hectometer equals 100 meters
- 1 decameter equals 10 meters

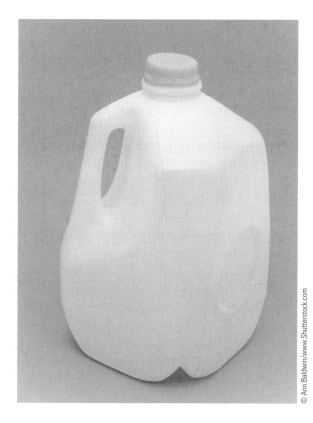

- 10 decimeters equal 1 meter
- 100 centimeters equal 1 meter
- 1,000 millimeters equal 1 meter

When measuring mass or weight:

- 1 kilogram equals 1,000 grams
- 1 hectogram equals 100 grams
- 1 decagram equals 10 grams
  - gram
    - 10 decigrams equal 1 gram
    - 100 centigrams equal 1 gram
    - 1,000 milligrams equal 1 gram

When measuring volume or liquid:

- 1 kiloliter equals 1,000 liters
- 1 hectoliter equals 100 liters
- 1 decaliter equals 10 liters
  - liter
    - 10 deciliters equal 1 liter
    - 100 centiliters equal 1 liter
    - 1,000 milliliters equal 1 liter

Because some parts of the world use English measurement and other parts use metric measurement, there will likely be both types of measurement on the products you buy and use, but sometimes you will have to convert one type of measurement to the other. In cases like these, a *conversion rate* is needed. A **conversion rate** is a rate that compares two measurements through division, with the intention of converting one measurement to another measurement. A **rate** compares two quantities through division. A rate can be written in several forms: whole numbers, fractions, decimals, and percentages.

For example, if you wanted to convert English measurement to metric measurement it would look like this:

- 1 gallon = 3.785 liters
- 1 pound = 453.59237 grams
- 1 mile = 1,600 meters

Or, if you wanted to convert metric measurement to English measurement, it would look like this:

- 1 liter = 0.264 gallons
- 1 gram = 0.00220462 pounds
- 1 meter = .000625 miles

Sometimes, when we work with measurement units and conversion rates, we may find that we need to use *cross multiplication*. **Cross multiplication** is a mathematical process that is used to compare two equivalent fractions when one of the fractions has an unknown value. Remember, we can find equivalent fractions by either multiplying or dividing the top and bottom of a fraction by the same number. For example:

$$\frac{3}{4} = \frac{3 \times 2}{4 \times 2} = \frac{6}{8} \text{ so therefore } \frac{3}{4} = \frac{6}{8}$$

There may also be instances when we will need to use a method for **converting multiple rates**, a conversion method that compares three or more measurement rates and through division and multiplication converts these differing measurements to one specific measurement rate.

Let's take a stab at measurements and converting measurements.

Note: Although these questions will sometimes require complicated calculations to reach the answer, we will go through each step to help you see all of the process when converting one type of measurement to another. In your everyday dealings, you may be able to find an easier way to come up with the answer you need; however, here we want you to see and understand how the answer is arrived at.

SHOW ME HOW

QUESTION 1: A 32-ounce (.9464-liter) bottle of conditioner cost $15.00. How much does the conditioner cost per ounce?

ANSWER: **STEP 1:** Consider the quantities that are needed for cost per ounce. Because we are looking for the cost per ounce, the quantities we need are the *cost* and the number of *ounces*.

    Cost = $15.00

    Ounces = 32

STEP 2: Set up a fraction to represent the rate. The numerator (top part of the fraction) will always be whatever measurement we desire. The denominator (bottom part of the fraction) will always be whatever it is we are comparing the desired measurement to.

$$\frac{\textit{Desired Measurement}}{\textit{Compared Measurement}} = \frac{\textit{Cost}}{\textit{Ounces}} = \frac{15.00}{32}$$

STEP 3: Perform any necessary operations to simplify the rate. Because all fractions are also division problems, we can simply divide the numerator by the denominator.

$$\frac{15.00}{32} = 15.00 \div 32$$

= .46875 or 47 cents per ounce.

STEP 4: Interpret the outcome.

For each ounce of conditioner we paid 47 cents. Therefore, if we purchased 64 ounces, we would expect to pay $30.00 (.46875 cents × 64).

QUESTION 2: If a liter of shampoo is approximately .2642 gallons, how many liters are equal to 10 gallons of shampoo?

ANSWER: **STEP 1:** Set up the two rates that will be needed to solve the problem. The rates must be equal so that we are comparing the same things.

1 Liter/.2642 gallons = unknown Liters/10 gallons

$$\frac{Desired\ Measurement}{Compared\ Measurement} = \frac{Desired\ Measurement}{Compared\ Measurement}$$

OR

$$\frac{1\ liter}{.264172\ gallons} = \frac{unknown\ liters}{10\ gallons}$$

OR

$$\frac{1}{.264172} = \frac{x}{10}$$

STEP 2: Cross multiply by multiplying a numerator (a number on the top) by a denominator (a number on the bottom). The numbers must be on opposite sides of the equal sign.

$$\frac{1}{.264172} = \frac{x}{10}$$

$$.264172x = 10 \times 1$$

$$.264172x = 10$$

STEP 3: Solve for x by treating the problem as an equation, which means we must isolate x by doing the opposite to .264172 of whatever is being done to x.

$$.264172x = 10$$

$$.264172x \div .264172 = 10 \div .264172\ (\textbf{Note:}\ \text{We must eliminate .264172.})$$

$$x = 37.8541253$$

STEP 4: Interpret and apply logic to the outcome.

$$\frac{1}{.264172} = \frac{x}{10}$$

$$\frac{1}{.264172} = \frac{37.8541253}{10}$$

37.8541253 liters is equal to 10 gallons of shampoo.

QUESTION 3: How many ounces of haircolor are in 1 milliliter?

ANSWER: **STEP 1:** Set up the rates that will be needed to solve the problem. Start with labels (words) to represent the rates so that we can apply logic to the mathematical process.

Note: The rates must move from one rate to the next rate, such as centiliters to liters, to gallons, to quarts, to pints, to cups, to ounces, unless there is a rate that will allow us to go from centiliters to ounces. We can create a rate that will go from gallons to ounces by simply multiplying 4 quarts by 2 pints by 2 cups by 8 ounces (4 × 2 × 2 × 8 = 128 *ounces* = 1 *gallon*). In our problem, we are looking for the ounces. Because the question states how many ounces are in 1 milliliter, we must end up with ounces, and because we are comparing ounces to milliliters, we will start with milliliters.

milliliter to *liters* to *gallons* to *ounces* = *ounces* per *milliliter*

OR

$$1 \times \frac{1\ liter}{1000\ millliters} \times \frac{1\ gallon}{3.785\ liters} \times \frac{128\ ounces}{1\ gallon} = \text{ounces per milliliter}$$

STEP 2: Perform any necessary operations to simplify the rates.

Note: Because all fractions are also division problems, we can divide the numerator by the denominator.

milliliters to liters to gallons to ounces = ounces per milliliter

$1 \times .001 \times .2642 \times 128 =$ ounces per milliliter

STEP 3: Combine the rates and multiply them.

milliliters to liters to gallons to ounces = ounces per milliliter

$1 \times .001 \times .2642 \times 128 = .0338176$

STEP 4: Interpret and apply logic to the outcome.

Our rate is .0038176 ounces per milliliter, and it means that 1 milliliter is the same as .0038176 ounces of haircolor.

CONVERTING MEASUREMENTS

There are many instances when you may need to convert an English measurement to a metric measurement or vice versa, but there will also be times when you need to convert measurements within each to a particular type of measurement. For example, you may go to the supply store to buy a gallon of shampoo because you know that your salon uses a gallon of shampoo per month. But there are no gallon sizes available, only quart bottles of shampoo. So, the question becomes, how many quarts will it take to equal a gallon of shampoo?

To make the conversion process easier, the following show two conversion tables: one for metric conversion and one for English conversion.

METRIC CONVERSION TABLE		
Distance	**Mass (Weight)**	**Volume(Liquid)**
1 kilometer = 1,000 meters	1 kilogram = 1,000 grams	1 kiloliter = 1,000 liters
1 hectometer = 100 meters	1 hectogram = 100 grams	1 hectoliter = 100 liters
1 decameter = 10 meters	1 decagram = 10 grams	1 decaliter = 10 liters
Meter	**Gram**	**Liter**
10 decimeters = 1 meter	10 decigrams = 1 meter	10 deciliters = 1 liter
100 centimeters = 1 meter	100 centigrams = 1 meter	100 centiliter = 1 liter
1,000 millimeters = 1 meter	1,000 milligrams = 1 meter	1,000 milliliter = 1 liter

© Milady, a part of Cengage Learning.

ENGLISH SYSTEM CONVERSION TABLE	
Distance	**Converting English to Metric**
12 inches = 1 foot	1 gallon = 3.785 liters
3 feet = 1 yard	1 pound = 453.59237 grams
1,760 yards = 1 mile	1 mile = 1,600 meters
Mass (Weight)	**Converting Metric to English**
16 oz = 1 pound	1 liter = 0.264 gallons
2,000 pounds = 1 ton	1 gram = 0.00220462 pounds
Volume (Liquid)	1 meter = 0.000625 miles
8 ounces = 1 cup	
2 cups = 1 pint	
2 pints = 1 quart	
4 quarts = 1 gallon	

© Milady, a part of Cengage Learning.

SHOW ME HOW

Using the two conversation tables shown previously, let's solve the following problems.

QUESTION 1: Convert 15.3 milliliters of developer to liters.

ANSWER: **STEP 1:** Determine how many places up or down we have to move in order to reach a liter. (**Note:** The metric system has a base of 10, which means as we move from one measurement to the next, we increase or decrease by multiples of 10. Because the decimal system is based on multiples of 10, we only have to move the decimal right or left based upon moving up or down the measurement chart.)

Liter ⟵ Ending Point
10 deciliters = 1 liter
100 centiliters = 1 liter
1,000 milliliters = 1 liter ⟵ Starting Point

From the starting point the move was 3 units up to the ending point

STEP 2: Because the move was 3 units up to reach a liter, the decimal must move 3 places to the left. We then fill in the empty place values with zeros.

Start	1st move	2nd move	3rd move	Answer
15.3	1.53	.153	.0153	.0153 Liters

15.3 milliliters of developer is equal to .0153 liters of developer.

QUESTION 2: Convert 7.3 kiloliters of styling lotion to centiliters.

ANSWER: **STEP 1:** Determine how many places up or down we have to move in order to reach a liter. (**Note:** The metric system has a base of 10, which means as we move from one measurement to the next, we increase or decrease by multiples of 10. Because the decimal system is based on multiples of 10, we only have to move the decimal right or left based upon moving up or down the measurement chart.)

1 kiloliter = 1,000 liters   ⟵——— Starting Point

1 hectoliter = 100 liters

1 decaliter = 10 liters

Liter

10 deciliters = 1 liter

100 centiliters = 1 liter   ⟵——— Ending Point

1,000 milliliters = 1 liter

From the starting point, the move was 5 units up to the ending point.

STEP 2: Because the move was 5 units down to reach a centiliter, the decimal must move 5 places to the right. We then fill in the empty place values with zeros.

Start	1st move	2nd move	3rd move	4th move	5th move	Answer
7.3	73.	730.	7,300.	73,000.	730,000.	730,000 centiliter

7.3 kiloliters of styling lotion is equal to 730,000 centiliters.

QUESTION 3: Convert 78 ounces of massage oil to gallons.

ANSWER: **STEP 1:** Determine the rates that must be used to convert ounces to gallons.

Ounces ⟶ Cups ⟶ Pints ⟶ Quarts ⟶ Gallons

$$78 \text{ ounces} \quad \frac{cups}{ounces} \quad \frac{pints}{cups} \quad \frac{quarts}{pints} \quad \frac{gallons}{quarts}$$

Note: Notice that the measurement that is desired is always the *numerator* (top part of the fraction), and the measurement that is being eliminated is always the *denominator* (bottom part of the fraction) in each rate.

STEP 2: Use the rates and multiplication to convert ounces to gallons.

$$78 \text{ ounces} \times \frac{1\,cup}{8\,ounces} \times \frac{1\,pint}{2\,cups} \times \frac{1\,quart}{2\,pints} \quad \frac{1\,gallon}{4\,quarts}$$

STEP 3: Use the cross-canceling method (a mathematical process that is used to simplify the multiplication of two or more fractions by allowing the division of any numerator and denominator by their greatest common factor or common measurement unit) to simplify the rates prior to performing multiplication

$$\frac{78\,\cancel{ounces}}{1} \times \frac{1\,\cancel{cup}}{8\,\cancel{ounces}} \times \frac{1\,\cancel{pint}}{2\,\cancel{cups}} \times \frac{1\,\cancel{quart}}{2\,\cancel{pints}} \quad \frac{1\,gallon}{4\,\cancel{quarts}}$$

STEP 4: Perform multiplication.

$$\frac{78 \div 2}{1} \times \frac{1}{8} \times \frac{1}{2 \div 2} \times \frac{1}{2} \times \frac{1\,gallon}{4} =$$

$$\frac{39 \times 1 \times 1 \times 1 \times 1\,gallon}{1 \times 8 \times 1 \times 2 \times 4} = \frac{39\,gallon}{64} = 39 \text{ gallons} \div 64 = .609375 \text{ gallons}$$

78 ounces of massage oil equals .609375 gallons.

QUESTION 4: Convert 3.28 gallons of disinfectant solution to pints.

ANSWER: **STEP 1:** Determine the rates that must be used to convert ounces to gallons.

Gallons $\longrightarrow$ Quarts $\longrightarrow$ Pints

3.28 gallons $\qquad \dfrac{quarts}{gallons} \qquad \dfrac{pints}{quarts}$

Note: Notice that the measurement that is desired is always the *numerator* (top part of the fraction), and the measurement that is being eliminated is always the *denominator* (bottom part of the fraction) in each rate.

STEP 2: Use the rates and multiplication to convert pints to gallons.

3.28 gallons $\qquad \dfrac{4 \; quarts}{1 \; gallons} \qquad \dfrac{2 \; pints}{1 \; quart}$

STEP 3: Use the cross-canceling method to simplify the rates prior to performing the multiplication.

$$\frac{3.28 \; \cancel{gallons}}{1} \times \frac{4 \; \cancel{quarts}}{1 \; \cancel{gallon}} \times \frac{2 \; pints}{1 \; \cancel{quart}}$$

STEP 4: Perform multiplication.

$$\frac{3.28}{1} \times \frac{4}{1} \times \frac{2 \; quarts}{1} = \frac{3.28 \times 4 \times 2 \; pints}{1 \times 1 \times 1} = \frac{26.24 \; pints}{1} = 26.24 \; pints$$

3.28 gallons of disinfectant solution is equal to 26.24 pints.

QUESTION 5: Convert 4 gallons of cleaning solution to milliliters.

ANSWER: **STEP 1:** Determine the rates that must be used to convert ounces to gallons.

Note: Notice that the measurement that is desired is always the *numerator* (top part of the fraction), and the measurement that is being eliminated is always the *denominator* (bottom part of the fraction) in each rate.

Gallons $\longrightarrow$ Liter $\longrightarrow$ Milliliters

4 gallons $\qquad \dfrac{liter}{gallons} \qquad \dfrac{milliliters}{liter}$

STEP 2: Use the rates and the multiplication operation to convert ounces to gallons.

4 gallons $\qquad \dfrac{1 \; liter}{.264 \; gallons} \qquad \dfrac{1,000 \; milliliters}{1 \; liter}$

STEP 3: Use the cross-canceling method to simplify the rates prior to performing the multiplication.

$$\frac{4 \; \cancel{gallons}}{1} \times \frac{1 \; \cancel{liter}}{.264 \; \cancel{gallons}} \times \frac{1,000 \; milliliters}{1 \cancel{liter}}$$

STEP 4: Perform the multiplication.

$$\frac{4 \div 4}{1} \times \frac{1}{.264 \div 4} \times \frac{1,000 \; milliliters}{1} = \frac{1 \times 1 \times 1,000 \; milliliters}{1 \times .066 \times 1} = \frac{1,000 \; milliliters}{.066}$$
$$= 15,151.5 \; milliliters$$

4 gallons of cleaning solution equals 15,151.5 milliliters.

QUESTION 6: Convert 17,830 milliliters of finger-waving lotion to pints.

ANSWER: **STEP 1:** Determine the rates that must be used to convert milliliters to pints.

Note: Notice that the measurement that is desired is always the *numerator* (top part of the fraction), and the measurement that is being eliminated is always the *denominator* (bottom part of the fraction) in each rate.

Milliliters $\longrightarrow$ Liter $\longrightarrow$ Gallons $\longrightarrow$ Quarts $\longrightarrow$ Pints

$$17830 \text{ milliliters} \quad \frac{liter}{milliliters} \quad \frac{gallons}{liter} \quad \frac{quarts}{gallons} \quad \frac{pints}{quart}$$

STEP 2: Use the rates and multiplication to convert milliliters to pints.

$$17830 \text{ milliliters} \times \frac{1 \text{ liter}}{1000 \text{ milliliters}} \times \frac{1 \text{ gallon}}{3.785 \text{ liter}} \times \frac{4 \text{ quarts}}{1 \text{ gallons}} \times \frac{1 \text{ pint}}{2 \text{ quarts}}$$

STEP 3: Use the cross-canceling method to simplify the rates prior to performing multiplication.

$$17830 \text{ milliliters} \times \frac{1 \text{ liter}}{1000 \text{ milliliters}} \times \frac{1 \text{ gallon}}{3.785 \text{ liters}} \times \frac{4 \text{ quarts}}{1 \text{ gallon}} \times \frac{1 \text{ pint}}{2 \text{ quarts}}$$

STEP 4: Perform the multiplication.

$$\frac{17830 \div 5}{1} \times \frac{1}{1000} \times \frac{1}{3.785 \div 5} \times \frac{4 \div 2}{1} \times \frac{1 \text{ quart}}{2 \div 2} = \frac{3566 \times 1 \times 1 \times 2 \times 1 \text{ pints}}{1 \times 1000 \times .757 \times 1 \times 1} = \frac{7132 \text{ quarts}}{757}$$

$$= 9.4214 \text{ pints}$$

17830 milliliters of finger waving lotion equals 9.4214 pints.

QUESTION 7: David purchased a 16-ounce tube of conditioner for $4.99. How much did David pay per milliliter for the 16-ounce tube of conditioner?

ANSWER: **STEP 1:** Determine the rates that must be used to convert the ounces to milliliters.

Volume (Liquid)
8 ounces = 1 cup
2 cups = 1 pint
2 pints = 1 quart
4 quarts = 1 gallon

Metric Conversion Table
1 kiloliter = 1,000 liters
1 hectoliter = 100 liters
1 decaliter = 10 liters
Liter
10 deciliters = 1 liter
100 centiliters = 1 liter
1,000 milliliters = 1 liter

Note: Some rates can be consolidated into one rate. For example, there are 8 ounces in a cup and 2 cups in a pint and 2 pints in a quart and 4 quarts in a gallon, so we could say:

8 ounces × 2 cups × 2 pints × 4 quarts × 1 gallon = 128 ounces = 1 gallon

Ounces $\longrightarrow$ Gallon $\longrightarrow$ Liters $\longrightarrow$ Milliliters

STEP 2: Use the rates and the multiplication operation to convert ounces to milliliters.

$$16 \text{ ounces} \times \frac{1 \text{ gallon}}{128 \text{ ounces}} \times \frac{3.785 \text{ liters}}{1 \text{ gallon}} \times \frac{1000 \text{ milliliters}}{1 \text{ liter}}$$

$$16 \div 16 \times \frac{1}{128 \div 16} \times \frac{3.785}{1} \times \frac{1000 \text{ milliliters}}{1}$$

$$= \frac{1 \times 1 \times 3.785 \times 1000 \text{ milliliters}}{1 \times 8 \times 1 \times 1}$$

$$\frac{3,785 \text{ milliliters}}{8} = 473.125 \text{ milliliters}$$

STEP 3: Divide the total price by the total milliliters to find the unit price.

$$\frac{Total\ price}{Total\ milliliters} = \text{unit price}$$

$$\frac{4.99}{473.125} = .010547 \text{ per milliliter}$$

David paid approximately 1cent per milliliter of conditioner.

QUESTION 8: Sophia can purchase a gallon of shampoo for $20 and liter bottles of the same shampoo for $7.50 each. Which purchase has the lowest unit price?

ANSWER: **STEP 1:** Convert both purchases to the same measurement unit. Convert gallons to liters or convert liters to gallons. It really doesn't matter. The problem can be solved either way.

Gallons $\longrightarrow$ Liters

$$1 \text{ Gallon} = \frac{liters}{gallons}$$

STEP 2: Use the rates and the multiplication operation to convert ounces to milliliters.

$$1 \text{ Gallon} \times \frac{3.785 \text{ liters}}{1 \text{ gallon}} = \frac{1 \times 3.785 \text{ liters}}{1} = 3.785 \text{ liters}$$

STEP 3: Divide the total price by the total milliliters to find the unit price.

$$\frac{Total\ price}{Total\ liters} = \text{unit price}$$

Unit Price for $20 Shampoo

$$\frac{20}{3.785} = 5.28404 \text{ per liter}$$
Unit Price = $5.28

Unit Price for $7.50 Shampoo

$$\frac{7.5}{1} = \$7.50 \text{ per liter}$$
Unit Price = $7.50

Note: The $20 shampoo was in gallons, so we needed a rate to convert it to liters. The $7.50 shampoo was already in liters; therefore, we did not need a rate to convert it because the $7.50 shampoo was already in the desired rate.

The $20 shampoo has the lowest unit price, which means that Sophia will save money by purchasing the $20 shampoo instead of the $7.50 shampoo.

QUESTION 9: If 128 ounces is equal to 1 gallon, how many ounces are equal to 5 gallons?

ANSWER: **STEP 1:** Determine the rate.

Ounces per gallon $\longrightarrow$ $\dfrac{ounces}{gallons}$

Note: Notice how the measurement that is desired (ounces) is the *numerator* (top part of the fraction), and the measurement that is being eliminated (gallons) is the *denominator* (bottom part of the fraction).

STEP 2: Compare the rates.

$$\frac{128\ ounces}{1\ gallon} = \frac{x\ ounces}{5\ gallons}$$

STEP 3: Use cross multiplication to find the unknown amount of ounces.

$$\frac{128\ ounces}{1\ gallons} \diagdown \frac{x\ ounces}{5\ gallons}$$

$128 \times 5 = 1x$

$640 = x$

640 ounces equal 5 gallons.

8–1 LET ME TRY

1. Convert 2.86 decagrams to centigrams.

2. Convert 36 centiliters to liters.

3. Convert 38 ounces to pints.

4. Convert 3.7 gallons to ounces.

5. Convert 3 gallons to liters.

6. Convert 823 liters to ounces.

1. Name the two types of measurements systems used today.

2. How does each system measure distance, mass, and volume?

3. What are the steps involved in converting an English measurement to a metric measurement?

4. What are the steps involved in converting a metric measurement to an English measurement?

Banking and Interest

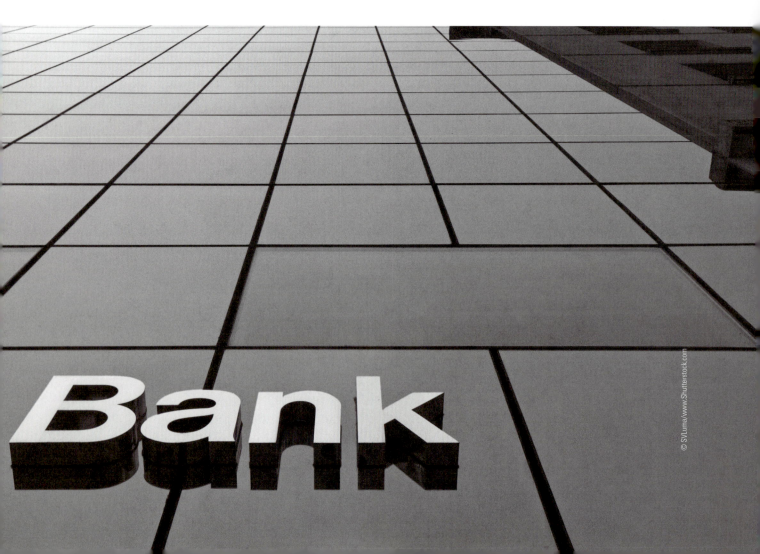

- Banking
- Interest

After completing this chapter, you will be able to:

1. Understand the difference between a beginning balance and an ending balance as indicated on a bank statement.

2. Explain the difference between principal and interest.

- amortization of a simple loan
- annual interest rate
- beginning balance
- compound period
- compounded interest
- compounding
- effective interest rate
- ending balance
- future value of compound interest
- future value of simple interest
- interest
- principal
- simple interest

S YOU HAVE ALREADY LEARNED, MANAGING YOUR CAREER AND RUNNING a business means that you have to have a handle on numbers, and a big part of "the numbers" has to do with banking, planning, budgeting, and interest. It is important to know how to read your bank statements, to understand your balances, fees, interest rates, and getting and paying off loans.

In this chapter we will take a look at banking practices, and particularly interest rates as they relate to bank accounts, borrowed monies, invested monies, and business credit cards.

BANKING

Anytime you consider your business—whether you realize it or not—your banking institution becomes your partner. It may be a silent partner, in that you may simply use it as a place to park monies in between transactions; or it can be an interactive partner, in that it could have loaned you money to invest in your business, and you have certain obligations to your bank as an investor in your business.

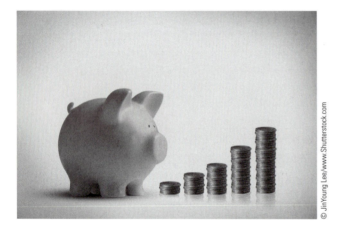

© JinYoung Lee/www.Shutterstock.com

Your relationship with your bank will be documented and recorded in the various statements you receive from the bank. On your bank statements you will find both a *beginning balance* and an *ending balance*.

A **beginning balance** is the amount of money the account has in it at the start of the period, which is usually a month. An **ending balance** is the amount of money the account has in it at the end of the month. A formula for how the ending balance is determined is: ending balance = beginning balance + deposits + other credits – (checks + withdrawals + bank charges).

SHOW **ME** HOW

QUESTION 1: What is this account's ending balance if all of the following numbers are correct for the account?

Beginning Balance:	$12,326.12
Deposits:	$16,728.59
Checks:	$ 11,710.00
Bank Charges:	$ 14.32
Withdrawals:	$ 1,382.43

ANSWER: **STEP 1:** Use the formula.

ending bank balance = beginning + deposits + other credits – (checks + withdrawals + bank charges)

STEP 2: Input the known values.

ending balance = $12,236.12 + 16,728.59 – (11,710 + 1,382.43 + 14.32)

STEP 3: Solve the problem by following the order of operations.

Ending Balance = 12,236.12 + 16,728.59 − (11,710 + 1,382.43 + 14.32)

Ending Balance = 12,236.12 + 16,728.59 − (13,106.75)

Ending Balance = 28,964.71 − 13,106.75

Ending Balance = 15,857.96

The account's ending balance is $15,857.96

INTEREST

Most bank accounts, whether they are checking or savings or some other longer-term account, pay interest. When you open an account at your bank, you are entering into an agreement with that bank. The agreement basically states that you will put your money in that institution, and until you need to use your money, you will allow the bank to use your money for loans or investments to its other customers. For allowing the bank to use your money that way, the bank pays you a fee, called **interest**.

The **compound period** is the amount of time it takes for interest paid on an account, which then becomes part of the principal and starts earning interest. The **principal** is the original monies put into the account. The faster the interest compounds, the more principal there is working to earn money.

Accounts that pay interest can have different compound periods. This addition of interest to the principal is called **compounding**.

The following are some examples of compound periods.

Daily: 365 times a year (every day)

Weekly: 52 weeks (every week)

Monthly: 12 times a year (every month)

Quarterly: 4 times a year (every 3 months)

Semiannually: 2 times a year (every 6 months)

Annually: 1 time a year (once a year)

A bank account, for example, may have its interest compounded every year—in this case, an account with $1,000 initial principal and 20% interest rate per year would have a balance of $1,200 at the end of the first year, and then $1,440 at the end of the second year, and so on.

Here is the formula for determining interest rate:

$$r = \frac{i}{p}$$

where

r = rate

i = interest paid

p = principal

Although you and your accountants will probably use special calculators to do all of the following calculations, it is important to understand the methodology behind what the numbers mean, so we will take you through each of the steps.

QUESTION 1: What is the interest rate if the following is true?

Interest paid (i): $1,230

Principal (p): $10,000

Rate (r) = ?

ANSWER: **STEP 1:** Use the formula.

$$r = \frac{i}{p}$$

STEP 2: Input the known values.

$$r = \frac{1,230}{10,000}$$

STEP 3: Solve the problem by following the order of operations.

$$r = \frac{1,230}{10,000} = 1,230 \div 10,000$$

$$r = .123 = 12.3\%$$

The interest rate on this account is 12.3%.

Types of Interest

The **annual interest rate** is the ratio of interest to principal before compounding any interest. The annual rate is also known as the *nominal rate.* Nominal means "in name only." Therefore the annual interest rate is the interest rate in name only. The annual interest rate is not the real interest rate, because the interest rate will change each time interest is compounded, creating a new rate called the *effective interest rate.*

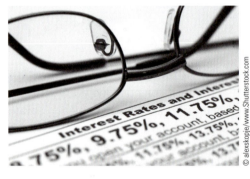

The **effective interest rate** is the ratio of interest to principal *after* compounding interest. The effective interest rate determines the real rate at which interest accrues. The formula for the effective interest rate is:

$$e = \left(1 + \frac{r}{n}\right)^n - 1$$

where

e = effective interest rate

n = compound period

QUESTION 1: If you have an account with an annual interest rate (r) of 8% and a compound period (n) that is daily (365 times a year), what will the effective interest rate (e) be?

ANSWER: **STEP 1:** Use the formula.

$$e = \left(1 + \frac{r}{n}\right)^n - 1$$

STEP 2: Input the known values.

$$e = \left(1 + \frac{.08}{365}\right)^{365} - 1$$

STEP 3: Solve the problem by following the order of operations.

$$e = \left(1 + \frac{.08}{365}\right)^{365} - 1$$

$$e = (1 + .000219)^{365} - 1$$

$$e = (1.000219)^{365} - 1$$

$$e = (1.08321) - 1$$

$$e = .08321 = 8.321\%$$

The effective interest rate is 8.321%.

Simple interest is the amount of money earned annually from principal or on a loan *without* compounding the interest. Simple interest is calculated using this formula:

$$i = p \times r \times t$$

SHOW ME HOW

QUESTION 1: Andre's account has $25,000 in principal (*p*), earns an annual interest rate (*r*) of 4.5%, and is locked in for 5 year's time (*t*). How much interest (*i*) will be paid on this account at the end of the 5 years?

ANSWER: **STEP 1:** Use the formula.

$$i = p \times r \times t$$

STEP 2: Input the known values.

$$i = 25,000 \times 4.5\% \times 5$$

STEP 3: Solve the problem by following the order of operations.

$$i = \$25,000 \times .045 \times 5$$

$$i = \$1,125 \times 5$$

$$i = \$5,625.00$$

Andre's account will earn $5,625 in interest over 5 years.

Compounded interest is the amount of money earned annually from principal or a loan and any past interest. The formula for compounded interest is:

$$i = p\left(1 + \frac{r}{n}\right)^{nt} - p$$

SHOW ME HOW

QUESTION 1: Marsha has $20,000 principal (*p*) in her account, and it earns an annual rate (*r*) of 5%, with a compound period (*n*) of quarterly (4 times a year). Two year's time (*t*) has passed since she put her money into that account. How much interest (*i*) has the account earned?

ANSWER: **STEP 1:** Use the formula.

$$i = p\left(1 + \frac{r}{n}\right)^{nt} - p$$

STEP 2: Input the known values.

$$i = 20{,}000 \left(1 + \frac{5\%}{4}\right)^{4 \times 2} - 20{,}000$$

STEP 3: Solve the problem by following the order of operations.

$$i = 20{,}000 \left(1 + \frac{.05}{4}\right)^{4 \times 2} - 20{,}000$$

$$i = 20{,}000 \left(1 + \frac{.05}{4}\right)^{4 \times 2} - 20{,}000$$

$$i = 20{,}000 \left(1 + .0125\right)^{4 \times 2} - 20{,}000$$

$$i = 20{,}000 \left(1.0125\right)^{4 \times 2} - 20{,}000$$

$$i = 20{,}000 \left(1.0125\right)^{8} - 20{,}000$$

$$i = 20{,}000 \times 1.10449 - 20{,}000$$

$$i = 22089.80 - 20{,}000$$

$$i = \$2{,}089.80$$

Marsha's account has earned $2,089.80 in 2 years.

The **future value of simple interest** is the value that money will be worth in the future, provided it is earning a specific, non-compound interest rate. The formula for this is:

Future value = Principal (1 + Annual rate × Time), or $Fv = p(1 + rt)$

SHOW ME HOW

QUESTION 1: Marty needs to know the future value (*Fv*) of his account if he invests $3,000 principal (*p*) for 5 year's time (*t*) at an annual interest rate of 6%.

ANSWER: **STEP 1:** Use the formula.
$Fv = p(1 + rt)$

STEP 2: Input the known values.
$Fv = 3{,}000(1 + 6\% \times 5)$

STEP 3: Solve the problem by following the order of operations.
$Fv = 3{,}000(1 + .06 \times 5)$
$Fv = 3{,}000(1 + .3)$
$Fv = 3{,}000 \times 1.3$
$Fv = \$3{,}900$

The future value of Marty's account after 5 years is $3,900.

Future value of compound interest is the value that money will be worth in the future provided it is earning a specific compound interest rate. The formula for this is:

$$Fv = p\left(1 + \frac{r}{n}\right)^{nt}$$

QUESTION 1: What is the future value (*Fv*) of an account continuing $5,000 in principal (*p*) and an annual rate (*r*) of 4% with a compound period (*n*) of twice a year (semiannually) for 6 years (*t*)?

ANSWER: **STEP 1:** Use the formula.

$$Fv = p\left(1 + \frac{r}{n}\right)^{nt}$$

STEP 2: Input the known values.

$$Fv = 5,000\left(1 + \frac{4\%}{2}\right)^{2 \times 6}$$

STEP 3: Solve the problem by following the order of operations.

$$Fv = 5,000\left(1 + \frac{.04}{2}\right)^{2 \times 6}$$

$$Fv = 5,000\left(1 + .02\right)^{2 \times 6}$$

$$Fv = 5,000\left(1.02\right)^{2 \times 6}$$

$$Fv = 5,000\left(1.02\right)^{12}$$

$$Fv = 5,000 \times 1.26824$$

$$Fv = \$6,341.21$$

The future value of an account containing $5,000 in principal with an annual rate of 4%, with a compound period (*n*) of twice a year for 6 years is $6,341.21.

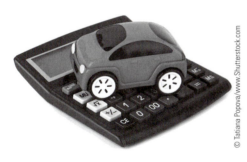

Have you ever borrowed money to buy a car, pay a mortgage, or go to school? **Amortization of a simple loan** is the process of repaying a loan with equal periodic payments. The formula for this is:

$$p = r\left[\frac{(1 + i)^{nt} - 1}{i\,(1 + i)^{nt}}\right] \text{ and } i = \frac{r}{n}$$

© Tatiana Popova/www.Shutterstock.com

QUESTION 1: Larry has taken a $10,000 loan (*p*) to pay for new salon equipment. The annual rate (*r*) of interest on the loan is 6%, and the compound period (*n*) is monthly for 10 year's time (*t*). How much will Larry's payment (*r*) be each month?

ANSWER: **STEP 1:** Use the formula.

$$i = \frac{r}{n}$$

$$p = r\left[\frac{(1 + i)^{nt} - 1}{i(1 + i)^{nt}}\right]$$

STEP 2: Input the known values.

$$i = \frac{.06}{12} = .005$$

$$10{,}000 = r\left[\frac{(1 + .005)^{12 \times 10} - 1}{.005(1 + .005)^{12 \times 10}}\right]$$

STEP 3: Solve the problem by following the order of operations.

$$10{,}000 = r\left[\frac{(1 + .005)^{12 \times 10} - 1}{.005(1 + .005)^{12 \times 10}}\right]$$

$$10{,}000 = r\left[\frac{(1.005)^{12 \times 10} - 1}{.005(1.005)^{12 \times 10}}\right]$$

$$10{,}000 = r\left[\frac{(1.005)^{120} - 1}{.005(1.005)^{120}}\right]$$

$$10{,}000 = r\left[\frac{1.819397 - 1}{.005 \times 1.819397}\right]$$

$$10{,}000 = r\left[\frac{.819397}{.009097}\right]$$

$$10{,}000 = r \times 90.0735$$

$$10{,}000 \div 90.0735 = r \times 90.0735 \div 90.0735 \text{ (eliminate the 90.0735)}$$

$$111.02 = r$$

Larry will make 120 monthly payments of $111.02. Thus, the future value (Fv) of the loan is $13,322.40. In other words, a $10,000 loan at 6% annual interest rate, compounded monthly for 10 years, costs $3,322.40 in interest.

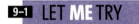

9-1 LET ME TRY

1. If a bank account has a beginning balance of $8,137.43, deposits of $10,346.31, checks of $6,531.21, bank charges of $39.86, and withdrawals of $561.39, how much is the ending balance?

2. If a bank account has a beginning balance of $19,749.41, checks of $10,563.83, bank charges of $41.37, other credits of $33.67, and an ending balance of $21,894.79, how much are the deposits?

3. Use the following information to find the annual interest rate.

   Interest paid (i) = $500

   Principal (p) = $8,000

   Rate (r) =?

4. Use the following information to find the simple interest rate.

Principal (p) = $10,000

Annual interest rate (r) = 7.25%

Time (t) = 5 years

Interest paid (i) = ?

5. Use the following information to find the future value of simple interest.

Future value (Fv) = ?

Principal (p) = $5,000

Annual interest rate (r) = 6%

Time (t) = 10 years

REVIEW QUESTIONS

1. Define and explain the difference between a beginning balance and an ending balance as indicated on a bank statement.

2. What is the difference between principal and interest?

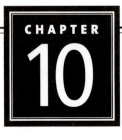

CHAPTER 10

Solving Problems Related to Inventory and Scheduling

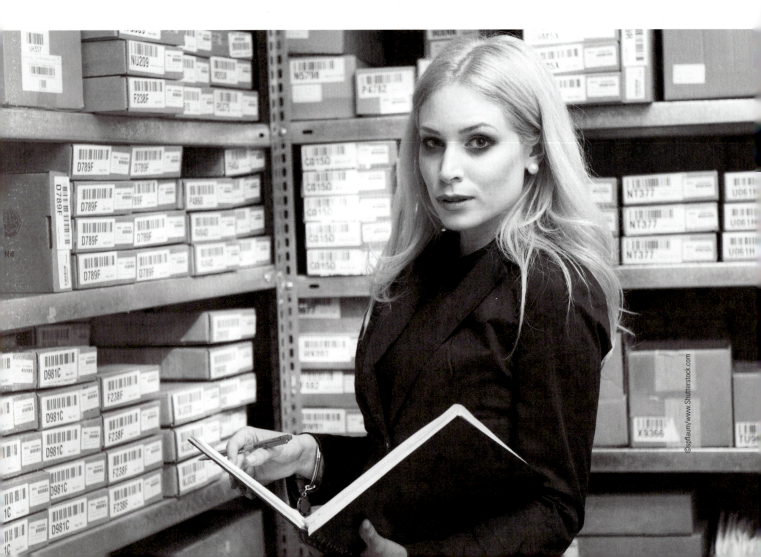

©spflaum/www.Shutterstock.com

- Inventory Management
- Time Management

LEARNING OBJECTIVES

After completing this chapter, you will be able to:

1. Define inventory.

2. Recognize the differences between periodic and perpetual inventory systems.

3. Identify the unit price of an item and how it is determined.

4. Define how time is measured in business, and name the four ways that time is tracked in a business setting.

5. Convert time from one form of measurement to another.

6. Know when to add, subtract, multiply, and divide time.

KEY TERMS

- administrative time
- converting time
- idle time
- inventory
- overlapping time
- periodic inventory system
- perpetual inventory system
- time
- unit price
- work time

Throughout this text, we have looked at how mathematics is an integral part of running and maintaining a successful salon and spa business. Even areas which we would not normally consider as based in mathematics have been impacted by our basic knowledge of math and how and why certain operations are useful. Two of those areas are scheduling and inventory control.

Although scheduling and inventory can be done manually, salon management software makes the task much easier. Most salon management software includes these features:

- **Appointment calendar** with walk-in appointment queue; a scheduling cancellation list resource; a waiting list; and appointment error-checking based upon space, equipment, and time available.

- **Client tracking** with client preference purchase patterns, target e-mail marketing, package creation and booking, fully integrated point-of-sale, service times, and individual pricing.

- **Inventory control** and tracking with one-step purchase orders.

Computer software in the salon also has vast marketing implications. The software tracks data about buying habits, names and addresses of clients, how often they come into the salon or spa—information which can be used to create customized promotions, e-mail alerts, coupons, and notices to clients.

Perhaps one of the greatest tools a salon software program provides is inventory control. In the fast-paced salon or spa, inventory, retail, and backbar products can be misused, misplaced, or depleted without too much notice initially, but the cost of this "missing" inventory can have disastrous results on the salon's bottom line.

Whether your salon or spa uses a computerized software program or not, you should have some knowledge of inventory control and practices and be comfortable tallying, adding, subtracting, and calculating the time spent in the salon and performing services. In this chapter, we will explore some of the basics.

INVENTORY MANAGEMENT

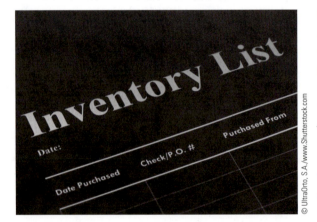

Inventory is a collection of supplies and products that a company uses to generate sales. There are two types of inventory systems: periodic and perpetual. A **periodic inventory system** is tracked by counting the inventory daily, weekly, or monthly, as you would with your backbar or service/treatment products. You need to be sure that when you leave the salon or spa at the end of the day, you have replenished supplies for the next day—so you will, in essence, take a quick inventory of what has been used. A **perpetual inventory system** is tracked administratively through purchase orders, sales invoices, and counting the inventory quarterly, semiannually, or annually. Perpetual inventory is how salons and spas account for products that they purchase in bulk, such as gallons of massage oil, cleansers, shampoos or conditioners, and how they inventory their retail-size products for sale to clients.

Perpetual Inventory List

Description	Beginning	Purchased	Used	Ending
Shampoo	6 gallons	3 gallons	_____	2 gallons
Conditioner	3 gallons	4 gallons	_____	1 gallon
Haircolor	10 @ 3 ounces	4 @ 3 ounces	_____	3 @ 3 ounces

© Milady, a part of Cengage Learning.

QUESTION 1: How many gallons of shampoo were used?

ANSWER: **STEP 1:** Use the formula.

Used = (Beginning + Purchased) − Ending

STEP 2: Input the known values.

Used = (6 + 3) − 2

STEP 3: Perform the math.

Used = (6 + 3) − 2

Used =   9 − 2

The salon used 7 gallons of shampoo.

QUESTION 2: How many tubes of haircolor were used?

ANSWER: **STEP 1:** Use the formula.

Used = (Beginning + Purchased) − Ending

STEP 2: Input the known values.

Used = (10 + 4) − 3

STEP 3: Perform the math.

Used = (10 + 4) − 3

Used =   14 − 3

The salon used 11 tubes of haircolor.

Another aspect of inventory has to do with unit pricing. **Unit price** is the amount that is paid for each unit. The formula for determine unit price is:

$$\text{Unit Price} = \frac{\textit{Total Price}}{\textit{Total Units}}$$

QUESTION 1: If 8 gallons of shampoo are purchased for a price of $151.84, how much is the unit price?

ANSWER: **STEP 1:** Use the formula.

$$\text{Unit Price} = \frac{\textit{Total Price}}{\textit{Total Units}}$$

STEP 2: Input the known values.

$$\text{Unit Price} = \frac{151.84}{8}$$

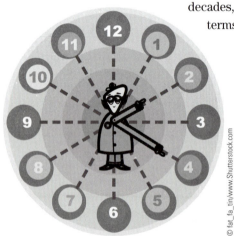

STEP 3: Perform the math.

Unit Price = $18.98 per gallon

QUESTION 2: If $164.28 of conditioner is purchased for a unit price of $13.69 per gallon, how many gallons were purchased?

ANSWER: **STEP 1:** Use the formula.

$$\text{Unit Price} = \frac{\text{Total Price}}{\text{Total Units}}$$

STEP 2: Input the known values.

$$13.69 = \frac{164.28}{\text{Total Units}}$$

STEP 3: Perform the math.

$$13.69 \,(\text{Total Units}) = \frac{164.28}{\cancel{\text{Total Units}}} \times \cancel{\text{Total Units}}$$

$$\frac{13.69 \;\text{Total Units}}{13.69} = \frac{164.28}{\cancel{13.69}}$$

$$13.69 \;\text{Total Units} = 164.28$$

$$\frac{164.28}{13.69} = 12$$

Total Units = 12 gallons

TIME MANAGEMENT

Time is a quantitative measurement that accounts for the initiation and expiration of all things. Time can be measured in increments of millenniums, centuries, decades, years, months, weeks, hours, minutes, and seconds. The following terms are units used in business tracking:

- **Idle time** is the time spent doing nothing.
- **Administrative time**, also known as *indirect labor*, is the time spent doing paperwork and making decisions.
- **Work time**, also known as *direct labor*, is the time directly related to rendering a service or selling a product to a client.
- **Overlapping time** is the time shared between two or more clients, such as completing a haircut while another client's haircolor processes.

Converting Time

Converting time is a process by which one measurement of time is changed to another measurement of time. This is an important concept, because we cannot add or subtract different units of measurement. Just like adding and subtracting fractions, there must be a conversion or change. Typically, we convert the larger unit to the smaller unit of measurement.

CONVERSION TABLE FOR UNITS OF TIME

12 months	=	1 year
7 days	=	1 week
52 weeks	=	1 year
24 hours	=	1 day
365 days	=	1 year
60 minutes	=	1 hour
5 days	=	1 business week
60 seconds	=	1 minute

© Milady, a part of Cengage Learning.

SHOW ME HOW

QUESTION 1: How many minutes are in a year?

ANSWER: **STEP 1:** Set up the rates that will be needed to solve the problem. Start with labels (words) to represent the rates so that logic can be applied to the mathematical process.

Note: The rates must move from one rate to the next rate (such as year to weeks to days to hours to minutes) unless there is a rate that will allow us to go straight from year to minutes. We are looking for the minutes because the question asks how many minutes are in a year. We must end up with minutes, and because we are comparing the minutes to a year, we will start with a year.

Year to days to hours to minutes = minutes per year

$$1 \text{ year} \times \frac{365 \text{ days}}{1 \text{ year}} \times \frac{24 \text{ hours}}{1 \text{ day}} \times \frac{60 \text{ minutes}}{1 \text{ hour}} = \text{minutes per year}$$

STEP 2: Perform any necessary operations to simplify the rates.

$$1 \cancel{\text{ year}} \times \frac{365 \cancel{\text{ days}}}{1 \cancel{\text{ year}}} \times \frac{24 \cancel{\text{ hours}}}{1 \cancel{\text{ day}}} \times \frac{60 \text{ minutes}}{1 \cancel{\text{ hour}}} = \text{minutes per year}$$

STEP 3: Combine the rates by multiplying them.

Year to days to hours to minutes = minutes per year

1 × 365 × 24 × 60 minutes = 525,600 minutes

STEP 4: Interpret and apply logic to the outcome.

Each year has 525,600 minutes in it.

Adding and Subtracting Time

When would you ever need to add or subtract time?

How often have you been in the situation where a client asks you, in the middle of her haircut or facial, if she can also have a brow wax? If you are doing your job well enough, it happens all of the time! Adding and subtracting time requires the combining of the same types of units of measurement.

SHOW ME HOW

QUESTION 1: If the average time to complete a haircolor is 75 minutes and the average time to complete a perm is $2\frac{1}{2}$ hours, what is the total time spent completing a haircolor and a perm?

ANSWER: STEP 1: Convert both measurements to the same unit of measurement.

Haircolor	+	Perm		= Total
75 minutes	+	$2\frac{1}{2}$ hours		= Total
75 minutes	+	$2\frac{1}{2}$ hours $\times \dfrac{60 \text{ minutes}}{1 \text{ hour}}$		= Total
75 minutes	+	$2\frac{1}{2}$ hours $\times \dfrac{60 \text{ minutes}}{1 \text{ hour}}$		= Total
75 minutes	+	$2\frac{1}{2} \times 60$ minutes		= Total
75 minutes	+	$2 \times 60 + \frac{1}{2} \times 60$ minutes		= Total
75 minutes	+	$120 + 30$ minutes		= Total
75 minutes	+	150 minutes		= Total

STEP 2: Perform the basic operations.

Haircolor	+	Perm	= Total
75 minutes	+	150 minutes	= Total
75 minutes	+	150 minutes	= 225 minutes

STEP 3: Once the units of measurement have been combined, they can be converted to any unit of measurement. In this case, convert the minutes to hours.

$$225 \text{ minutes} \times \frac{1 \text{ hour}}{60 \text{ minutes}} = \frac{225 \text{ hours}}{60} = 3.75 \text{ hours}$$

The total time spent performing the haircolor and the perm is 3.75 hours.

QUESTION 2: Danny has a 3-hour time slot scheduled for Mrs. Teeny, and she has asked for a haircut and color. If she also wants to have an upper lip waxing, which will take 20 minutes, how much time will Danny have to complete her cut and color service?

ANSWER: STEP 1: Convert both measurements to the same unit of measurement.

Cut and Color	−	Waxing	= Total
3 hours	−	20 minutes	= Total
3 hours $\times \dfrac{60 \text{ minutes}}{1 \text{ hour}}$	−	20 minutes	= Total
3 hours $\times \dfrac{60 \text{ minutes}}{1 \text{ hour}}$	−	20 minutes	= Total
3×60 minutes	−	20 minutes	= Total
180	−	20 minutes	= Total

STEP 2: Perform the basic operations.

Cut and Color	–	Waxing	= Total
180	–	20 minutes	= Total
180	–	20 minutes	= 160

STEP 3: Once the units of measurement have been combined, they can be converted to any unit of measurement.

minutes   to   hours

$$160 \text{ minutes} \times \frac{1 \text{ hour}}{60 \text{ minutes}} = \frac{160 \text{ hours}}{60} = 2.66 \text{ hours}$$

Danny will have 2.66 hours (or 2 hours and 40 minutes) to complete Mrs. Teeny's cut and color service.

Multiplying Time

Multiplying time is the process of combining sets of the same unit of measurement. Because we are combining the same units, there is no need to convert the units, because they are already the same.

QUESTION 1: If David has completed half of a haircolor service and has 3 more haircolor services to complete, how much more time will he have to spend on haircoloring if the average haircolor takes 75 minutes to complete?

ANSWER: **STEP 1:** Set up a table to illustrate what steps are required to solve the problem.

Time spent on haircolor	×	Quantity	= Total time
75 minutes	×	$3\frac{1}{2}$	= Total time

STEP 2: Perform the multiplication.

75 minutes	×	$3\frac{1}{2}$	= Total time
75 minutes	×	3.5	= Total time
75 minutes	×	3.5	= 262.5 minutes

STEP 3: Once the units of measurement have been combined, they can be converted to any unit of measurement.

minutes   to   hours

$$262.5 \text{ minutes} \times \frac{1 \text{ hour}}{60 \text{ minutes}} = \frac{262.5 \text{ hours}}{60} = 4.375 \text{ hours}$$

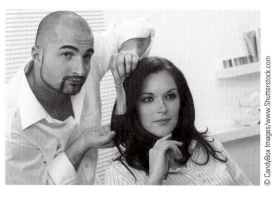

Hours	Minutes	Seconds
4.375	60 × .375 = 22.5	60 × .5 = 30
4 hours	22 minutes	30 seconds

David will need to spend an additional 4 hours, 22 minutes, and 30 seconds performing haircolor services to complete all of his haircolor appointments.

Dividing Time

Dividing time is the process of subtracting sets of the same unit of measurement. Since we are subtracting the same units, there is no need to convert the units because they are already the same.

QUESTION 1: If the average time spent on each client is 1 hour and 15 minutes and there are 50 business hours in a week, how many clients can be serviced in 1 week?

STEP 1: Convert the units to the same measurement of time.

Business hours in a week	÷	Time on each client
50 hours	÷	1 hour and 15 minutes
50 hours	÷	$1 \text{ hour and } \left(15 \text{ minutes} \times \dfrac{1 \text{ hour}}{60 \text{ minutes}}\right)$
50 hours	÷	$1 \text{ hour and } \left(15 \text{ minutes} \times \dfrac{1 \text{ hour}}{60 \text{ minutes}}\right)$
50 hours	÷	$1 \text{ and } \dfrac{15}{60} \text{ hours}$
50 hours	÷	1.25 hours

STEP 2: Perform the division.

50 ÷ 1.25

5000 ÷ 125 (move the decimal two places to the right) = 40

STEP 3: Apply logic to the answer.

40 is the number of clients that can be serviced each week at 1.25 hours a client, equaling a total of 50 hours for all 40 clients.

QUESTION 2: If David's appointment sheet states that he has 2 haircolor services scheduled at 75 minutes each, and 3 perm services scheduled at 2 hours for each, what time will David finish work that day, if he starts at 9 a.m. and does not take a lunch break?

ANSWER: **STEP 1:** Convert both measurements to the same unit of measurement.

Perms	+	Haircolor	= Total
2 hours	+	75 minutes	= Total
$2 \text{ hours} \times \dfrac{60 \text{ minutes}}{1 \text{ hour}}$	+	75 minutes	= Total
$2 \text{ hours} \times \dfrac{60 \text{ minutes}}{1 \text{ hour}}$	+	75 minutes	= Total
$2 \times 60 \text{ minutes}$	+	75 minutes	= Total
120 minutes	+	75 minutes	= Total

STEP 2: Perform the basic operations

Perms	+	Haircolor	= Total
3 @ 120 minutes	+	2 @ 75 minutes	= Total
360 minutes	+	150 minutes	= 510 minutes

STEP 3: Once the units of measurement have been combined, they can be converted to any unit of measurement

minutes   to   hours

$$510 \text{ minutes } \times \frac{1 \text{ hour}}{60 \text{ minutes}} = \frac{510 \text{ hours}}{60} = 8.5 \text{ hours}$$

STEP 4: Interpret and apply logic to the outcome.

Time	Hours Worked
9 a.m. to 12 p.m.	3 hours
12 p.m. to 5 p.m.	5 hours
5 p.m. to 5:30 p.m.	.5 hours (.5 hours × 60 minutes = 30 minutes)

David will finish at 5:30 p.m. if he starts at 9 a.m. and does not take a lunch break.

QUESTION 3: Sarah has a very, very busy day booked. She knows that she will have to work late, but she isn't quite sure how long all of the services will take. She is booked for 10 waxing services with an average time of 20 minutes each; 5 shaves with an average time of 35 minutes each; and 2 perms with an average time of $2\frac{1}{2}$ hours each. How many hours will Sarah work today?

STEP 1: Set up a table to illustrate what steps are required to solve the problem.

Time Spent on each service	×	Quantity	= Total time
Waxing: 20 minutes	×	10	= Total time
Shaves: 35 minutes	×	5	= Total time
Perms: $2\frac{1}{2}$ hours (2.5 × 60)	×	2	= Total time

(**Note:** Convert the $2\frac{1}{2}$ hours to minutes by multiplying $2\frac{1}{2}$ by 60 = 150 minutes. Each hour has 60 minutes in it; therefore, the first hour has 60 minutes, and the second hour has 60 minutes, and the half an hour only has 30 minutes in it.)

STEP 2: Perform the multiplication.

Waxing	20 minutes × 10	= 200 minutes
Shaves	35 minutes × 5	= 175 minutes
Perms	150 minutes × 2	= 300 minutes
Total minutes		= 675 minutes

STEP 3: Once the units of measurement have been combined, they can be converted to any unit of measurement.

minutes   to   hours

$$675 \text{ minutes } \times \frac{1 \text{ hour}}{60 \text{ minutes}} = \frac{675 \text{ hours}}{60} = 11.25 \text{ hours or } 11\frac{1}{4} \text{ hours}$$

Sarah will work $11\frac{1}{4}$ hours today (or 11 hours and 15 minutes).

1. Use the information below to determine how much shampoo, conditioner, and 3-ounce tubes of haircolor were used.

Description	Beginning	Purchased	Used	Ending
Shampoo	4 gallons	3 gallons	_____	1 gallon
Conditioner	6 gallons	3 gallons	_____	4 gallons
Haircolor	6 @ 3 ounces	2 @ 3 ounces	_____	4 @ 3 ounces

2. Use the information below to determine how much shampoo, conditioner, and 3-ounce tubes of haircolor should be left at the end of the month.

Description	Beginning	Purchased	Used	Ending
Shampoo	4 gallons	6 gallons	5 gallons	_____
Conditioner	3 gallons	5 gallons	6 gallons	_____
Haircolor	5 @ 3 ounces	4 @ 3 ounces	6 @ 3 ounces	_____

3. How many seconds are there in 7.5 hours?

4. How many hours are there in 480 minutes?

5. How many weeks are in 154 days?

6. If Arlene's calendar shows that she has 1 haircolor scheduled today, which will take 75 minutes, and 5 perms scheduled at 2.25 hours for each, at what time will Arlene finish if she starts at 8 a.m.?

7. If David performed 6 haircuts with an average time of 25 minutes each, 8 shaves with an average time of 30 minutes each, and 3 perms with an average time of $2\frac{1}{4}$ hours each, how many hours did he spend all together on the haircuts, shaves, and perms?

1. What is inventory, and why is it useful to track it carefully?

2. Define periodic and perpetual inventory systems, and describe which types of products in a salon or spa may be tracked by each method.

3. What is an item's unit price and how is it determined?

4. How is time defined? Name the four types of time that are tracked in a business setting.

5. What are the general steps involved in converting time from one form of measurement to another form of measurement?

6. On Tuesday John is booked for 1 hour on a haircolor, $1\frac{1}{2}$ hours styling an updo, and 45 minutes on a haircut. How long will John spend in the salon on Tuesday?

7. Andy has a doctor's appointment on Friday and plans on using 4 personal hours so he can go to the doctor. If he usually works 5 days in the salon, how many days will Andy work that week?

8. Bonnie has 2 hours open on Saturday, when a client calls to book two facials for Saturday. Each facial is 75 minutes long. Can Bonnie accommodate the request?

9. Amy has 3 free hours and donates that time to a shelter for homeless children. It takes her 40 minutes to complete 1 haircut, so how many haircuts can she perform in 3 hours during her time at the homeless shelter?

Appendix 1: Metric Conversion Tables

Conversion Formula for Inches to Centimeters: (number of) inches × 2.54 = centimeters

LENGTH	
Inches	**Centimeters**
1/8 inch (.125 inches)	0.317 centimeters
1/4 inch (.25 inches)	0.635 centimeters
1/2 inch (.50 inches)	1.27 centimeters
3/4 inch (.75 inches)	1.9 centimeters
1 inch	2.54 centimeters
2 inches	5.1 centimeters
3 inches	7.6 centimeters
6 inches	15.2 centimeters
12 inches	30.5 centimeters

© Milady, a part of Cengage Learning.

Conversion Formula for U.S. Fluid Ounces to Milliliters: (amount of) U.S. fluid ounce (fl. oz.) × 29.573 milliliters (ml)

Conversion Formula for U.S. Fluid Ounces to Liters: (amount of) U.S. fluid ounce (fl. oz.) × .029573 liters (l)

VOLUME (LIQUID)	
U.S. Fluid Onces	**Milliliters/liters**
1 fluid ounce (1/8 cup)	29. 57 milliliters/.02957 liters
2 fluid ounces (1/4 cup)	59.14 milliliters/.05914 liters
4 fluid ounces (1/2 cup)	118.29 milliliters/.11829 liters
6 fluid ounces (3/4 cup)	177.43 milliliters/.17743 liters
8 fluid ounces (1 cup)	236.58 milliliters/.23658 liters
16 fluid ounces (1 pint)	473.16 milliliters/.47316 liters
32 fluid ounces (1 quart)	946.33 milliliters/.94633 liters
33.81 fluid ounces (1 liter)	1,000 milliliters/1 liter
64 fluid ounces (1/2 gallon)	1,892.67 milliliters/1.8926 liters
128 fluid ounces (1 gallon)	3,785.34 milliliters/3.78534 liters

© Milady, a part of Cengage Learning.

Conversion Formula for Degrees Fahrenheit (°F) to Degrees Celsius (°C): °C = (°F-32) × (5/9) ***

TEMPERATURE	
Degrees Fahrenheit (°F)	**Degrees Celsius (°C)**
32°	0°
40°	4.444°
50°	10°
60°	15.556°
70°	21.111°
80°	26.667°
98.6°	37°
200°	93.333°
300°	148.889°
400°	204.444°

*** If you have a Fahrenheit temperature of 40 degrees and you want to convert it into degrees on the Celsius scale: Using the conversion formula, first subtract 32 from the Fahrenheit temperature of 40 degrees to get 8 as a result. Then multiply 8 by five and divide by nine (8 × 5)/9 to get the converted value of 4.444 degrees Celsius.

Appendix 2: Answer Key to Review Questions & Let Me Try

CHAPTER 1
Review Questions

1. Define mathematics and name the four mathematical operations used in problem-solving.
ANSWER: Mathematics is a universal language that is expressed with numbers, graphs, shapes, symbols, and signs of operations. The four operations used in problem-solving are addition, subtraction, multiplication, and division.

2. In the equation $7 + 2 = 9$, which number(s) represents the addends and which number(s) represents the sum?
ANSWER: In the equation $7 + 2 = 9$, 7 and 2 represent the addends and 9 represents the sum.

3. List the key words within a problem that indicate addition is the proper operation to use to solve it.
ANSWER: The key words within a problem that indicate addition is the proper operation to use to solve the problem are *all*, *total*, *increase* or *increased*, and *sum*.

4. In the equation $9 - 2 = 7$, which number(s) represents the minuend, which number(s) represents the subtrahend, and which number(s) represents the difference?
ANSWER: In the equation $9 - 2 = 7$, 9 represents the minuend, 2 represents the subtrahend, and 7 represents the difference.

5. List the key words within a problem that indicate subtraction is the proper operation to use to solve it.
ANSWER: The key words within a problem that indicate subtraction is the proper operation to use to solve a problem are *change*, *less than*, *decreased*, and *difference*.

6. In the equation $3 \times 2 = 6$, which number(s) represents the factors and which number(s) represents the product?
ANSWER: In the equation $3 \times 2 = 6$, 3 and 2 represent the factors and 6 represents the product.

7. List the key words within a problem that indicate multiplication is the proper operation to use to solve it.
ANSWER: The key words within a problem that indicate multiplication is the proper operation to use to solve a problem are *per*, *total*, *factors*, *twice*, *times*, and *product*.

8. In the equation $6 \div 2 = 3$, which number(s) represents the dividend, which number(s) represents the divisor, and which number(s) represent the quotient?
ANSWER: In the equation $6 \div 2 = 3$, 6 represents the dividend, 2 represents the divisor, and 3 represents the quotient.

9. List the key words within a problem that indicate division is the proper operation to use to solve it.
ANSWER: The key words within a problem that indicate division is the proper operation to use to solve a problem are *cost per unit*, *each*, *per*, or *quotient*.

10. Name at least three ways beauty and wellness professionals can use the four mathematical operations in their every day work.
ANSWER: Three ways a beauty and wellness professional can use the four mathematical operations in their everyday work are: 1) to determine the number of hours available for them to work; 2) to determine the

number of services and treatments they can provide in their work schedule; and 3) to determine promotional pricing and discounts for products they may need to purchase.

11. What is an opposite number? Give an example of how it can be useful.
ANSWER: An opposite number is the number's reciprocal, the inverted form of the number where the top part of the number and bottom part of the number change places when written in fraction form. Opposite numbers can be useful when you must, for example, determine monies that may be owed but have not yet been paid out of monies earned.

12. Define and explain the associative property.
ANSWER: The associative property is a property that is used with addition or multiplication but not both at the same time. The property states that the grouping of the numbers in an equation in different arrangements will not affect the answer. For example: $3 + (4 + 5) = 12$ and $(3 + 4) + 5 = 12$ are equal.

13. Define and explain the commutative property.
ANSWER: The commutative property is used with addition or multiplication but not both at the same time. The commutative property states that moving the numbers around, changing the order of the numbers, will not affect the answer. For example:
$3 + 4 + 5 = 12$ and $5 + 4 + 3 = 12$ are equal.

14. Define and explain the distributive property.
ANSWER: The distributive property is a property that is used with multiplication, addition, and subtraction. Multiplication and at least one of the other operations must be present. The distributive property states that we multiply the number on the outside of the parentheses by everything that is on the inside of the parentheses, completing the operation in the parentheses first. For example: $4 \times (\$25 + \$35) = \$240$.

15. Define and explain the identity property.
ANSWER: The identity property is a property that is used with addition or multiplication and it states that when zero is added to a number or when a number is multiplied by 1 it will not change the original number. For example: $8 + 0 = 8$ and $8 \times 1 = 8$.

16. Define and explain the inverse property.
ANSWER: The inverse property is a property that is used with addition or multiplication. It states that any time you add a number to its opposite the answer is zero. For example: $8 + (-8) = 0$. Any time you multiply a number by its reciprocal (opposite) the answer is 1. For example: $8 \times \frac{1}{8} = 1$.

Let Me Try

LET ME TRY 1–1
1. Talia ordered 6 tubes of haircolor on Monday and 4 tubes of haircolor on Friday. How many tubes of haircolor did she order in total?
ANSWER: $6 + 4 = 10$
2. Jason purchased 3 items. The first cost $312, the second cost $289, and the third cost $154. How much did he have to pay for all three items?
ANSWER: $\$312 + \$289 + \$154 = \$755$

LET ME TRY 1–2
1. A bottle of hair conditioner cost $6, and Maria paid the clerk with a $10 bill. How much change should Maria receive?
ANSWER: $\$10 - \$6 = \$4$

2. Joy charged Brenda $85 for a massage, and Brenda paid Joy with a $100 bill. How much money should be returned to Brenda?
ANSWER: $100 − $85 = $15

LET ME TRY 1–3
1. Maylie purchased 6 bottles of nail polish for $5 each. What is the total of the 6 bottles of polish at $5 each?
ANSWER: $6 \times \$5 = \$30$
2. Ally purchased 6 boxes of foundation for $24 per box. How much did Ally pay for all the boxes of foundation?
ANSWER: $\$24 \times 6 = \$144$

LET ME TRY 1–4
1. Lisa paid $100 for 5 bulbs for her laser hair-removal machine. What is the quotient of the $100 cost and the 5 bulbs?
ANSWER: $\$100 \div 5 = \$20$
2. One day Allen is offered a promotional deal from his supplier. If he is willing to buy 4 cases of shampoo, the supplier will sell all 4 cases for $112 instead of the regular price of $35 per case. If Allen agrees to buy all 4 cases, how much will he pay for each case? What will his per case savings be?
ANSWER: $\$112 \div 4 = \$28$ (promotional price per case) $35 (regular price per case) − $28 (promotional price per case) = $7 (savings per case)

LET ME TRY 1–5
1. What is the opposite of 8?
ANSWER: The opposite of 8 is −8.
2. What is the **o**pposite of −5?
ANSWER: The opposite of −5 is 5.
3. What is the reciprocal of $\frac{7}{1}$?
ANSWER: The **r**eciprocal of $\frac{7}{1}$ is $\frac{1}{7}$.
4. What is the reciprocal of $\frac{8}{12}$?
ANSWER: The reciprocal of $\frac{8}{12}$ is $\frac{12}{8}$.

LET ME TRY 1–6
1. If Jane does inventory on Tuesday, and that same day she orders 7 tubes of haircolor in one phone call and then calls back to order 3 bottles of acetone and 4 jars of polymer powder, how many items did Jane order for her spa?
ANSWER: $7 + (3 + 4) = 14$
2A. Marty is seeing 5 clients today, and each of them is having a haircut that costs $25 and a color service that costs $45. How much will Marty's services total?
ANSWER: $5 \times (\$25 + \$45) = \$350$
2B. If Marty can successfully upsell 2 of his clients and recommends that they purchase a duo of color-enhancing shampoo and conditioner for $25, how much will his sales total?
ANSWER: $3 \times (\$25 + \$45)$ (clients with no retail purchase) $+ 2 \times (\$25 + \$45 + \$25)$ (clients with a retail purchase = $3 \times (\$70) = \$210$ plus $2 \times (\$95) = \$190 = \$400$ total

LET ME TRY 1–7
1A. Barry goes to the supply store and picks up a shampoo cape ($12.99), a dozen of styling combs ($6.99), and a bottle of haircolor ($3.25). He goes to check out and the clerk rings them up. What is his total?
ANSWER: $\$12.99 + \$6.99 + \$3.25 = \$23.23$
1B. If Barry had purchased the very same items as above but the check-out clerk had rung up the bottle of haircolor first, then the dozen styling combs, and finally the shampoo cape, how much would Barry's total have been?
ANSWER: $\$3.25 + \$6.99 + \$12.99 = \$23.23$

1A. On Monday morning Gina has 2 UV gel nail services scheduled. She will charge $35 for each. On Monday afternoon she has 3 manicures and a pedicure scheduled, for which she charges $25 for the manicures and $30 for the pedicure. How much will her services total on Monday?

ANSWER: $2 \times (\$35) + 3 \times (\$25) + 1 \times (\$30) = \$175$

1B. On Tuesday morning, Gina is scheduled to perform 3 manicures at $25 each, and a pedicure at $30, and in the afternoon she is scheduled to perform 2 polymer powder and monomer liquid nail enhancement services for $35 each. How much will her service total on Tuesday? Did Gina make more money on Monday or Tuesday?

ANSWER: $3 \times (\$25) + 1 \times (\$30) + 2 \times (\$35) = \$175$. Gina made the same amount of money on each day.

2A. The Derma Brilliance Spa is running a special. If a client brings in the postcard that was mailed to them, they get $10 off of any service that costs $50 or more. The estheticians are excited because the postcard mailer has generated lots of interest and their schedules are full. Monica's schedule indicates that she has 4 clients that day and each is booked for a 1½-hour facial, priced at $80. How much will Monica's service total be?

ANSWER: $4 \times (\$80 - \$10) = \$280$

2B. If Monica also recommends a paraffin wax treatment to her clients, which costs an additional $22, and two of her clients agree to have it, how much will Monica's total be now?

ANSWER: $2 \times (\$80 - \$10) + 2 \times (\$80 + \$22 - \$10) = \$324$

1. Patty has advertised her new salon in the local newspaper for the first time. In the ad it says that if the client mentions reading about the salon in the newspaper, she will receive a 25% savings on her services that day. Patty has seen 5 clients since the ad has run, but none have mentioned the ad. How many clients has she seen?

ANSWER: 5 clients + 0 ad mentions = 5 clients

2. Tim has decided that he needs to hire a full-time receptionist instead of relying on stylists to answer the phone, make appointments, and help clients. He has enough money to hire 1 receptionist for the 52 weeks of the upcoming year. How many weeks will his salon have a receptionist?

ANSWER: 52 weeks × 1 receptionist = 52 weeks

1. Anton ordered 24 tubes of spiking glue at the beginning of the week, and by the end of the week he realizes that he has sold 12 tubes of spiking glue and that 3 tubes were returned to the salon for a refund because they were leaking and gooey. How many tubes of spiking glue does Anton have on hand to sell?

ANSWER: $24 - 12 = 12 + -3 = 9$

CHAPTER 2
Review Questions

1. Why is it important to a salon or spa professional to efficiently schedule clients and appointments?

ANSWER: It is important for a salon or spa professional to efficiently schedule clients and appointments because scheduling is the lifeblood of the salon and spa business—it is the schedule through which the revenue stream comes into and goes out of the business. So scheduling smartly is an imperative goal. Making the best, wisest use of the schedule while at work is one good way to ensure that your business remains financially secure.

2. What are integers, and how are they used in the appointment scheduling process?

ANSWER: Integers are positive or negative whole numbers like 1, 2, and 3 which are positive numbers and −1, −2, −3 and so forth which are negative numbers. In appointment scheduling, positive numbers are viewed as hours that are available for scheduling while negative numbers are considered as used hours.

3. What are fractions, and how are they used in the appointment scheduling process?

ANSWER: Fractions count a portion or piece of something; a fraction is a ratio that compares two numbers by division. There is a top and a bottom number for every fraction, written as $\frac{1}{2}$ for example. Since we want to make the best use of our time in a day and because not every service takes exactly 1 hour to complete, fractions are important in scheduling for efficiency so that valuable time is not wasted.

4. What are the most important rules for adding integers? How can they help you in appointment planning?

ANSWER: There are two important rules for adding integers; they are: 1) When adding integers, if the numbers have the same sign, add the numbers and attach the sign of the larger digit. This is called the *same sign sum*. 2) When adding integers that have different signs, find the difference between (subtract) the numbers and attach the sign of the larger digit. This is called the *different sign difference*. Knowing these rules can help you in appointment planning because they will help you to realize how much actual time is available for scheduling clients and services.

5. What are the most important rules for subtracting integers? How can they help you in appointment planning?

ANSWER: There is one important rule for subtracting integers: Never subtract negative integers. Change the subtraction sign to addition, then change the sign of the number following the addition sign to its opposite and last, but not least, follow the rule for adding integers with the same signs or different signs. This rule is helpful in appointment planning because it is impossible to subtract time from a negative number.

6. What are the most important rules for multiplying integers? How can they help you in appointment planning?

ANSWER: There is one important rule for multiplying integers: If the signs are different in the problem, the answer is negative and if the signs are the same in the problem, the answer is positive. Knowing whether an answer is positive or negative allows us to know how much time is actually available to spend with clients.

7. What are the most important rules for dividing integers? How can they help you in appointment planning?

ANSWER: Division of integers employs the same rule that multiplication of integers employs: If the signs are different in the problem, the answer is negative and if the signs are the same in the problem, the answer is positive. Sometimes you will need to find the difference between certain numbers or you will need to know how much time may be left in your schedule for making appointments—in which case division can make all the difference.

Let Me Try

LET ME TRY 2–1

1. $5 + -7 = -2$
2. $-5 + 7 = 2$
3. $-5 + -7 = -12$
4. $5 + 7 = 12$

LET ME TRY 2–2

1. $7 \times (-5) = -35$
2. $(-7) \times (-5) = 35$
3. $35 \div (-7) = -5$
4. $(-35) \div (-7) = 5$

CHAPTER 3
Review Questions

1. What is a fraction? Give three examples of fractions.

ANSWER: A fraction is a ratio (the relationship in quantity, amount, or size between two or more things) that compares two numbers by dividing one into the other. A fraction is a division problem waiting to happen. There is a top and a bottom number for every fraction. Three examples of fractions are: $\frac{1}{5}, \frac{3}{4}, \frac{5}{12}$.

2. How are fractions simplified? Why is this useful in inventory management?

ANSWER: Fractions are simplified by reducing large numbers by dividing the numerator and the denominator of a fraction by the same number. This is useful in inventory management because working with fractions larger than $\frac{1}{2}$ or $\frac{2}{3}$ is difficult and cumbersome. Simplifying fractions also allows us to add and subtract fractions so that we can get inventory totals.

3. Describe what an equivalent fraction is and give three examples.

ANSWER: An equivalent fraction is when two fractions look different but have the same value and are obtained when we either multiply or divide the numerator and the denominator of a fraction by the same number. Some examples of equivalent fractions are: $\frac{1}{2}, \frac{2}{4}$, and $\frac{3}{6}$.

4. Describe the process for adding fractions with like denominators.

ANSWER: When two fractions have like denominators, you can add them by adding the top numbers together and putting their sum over the denominator. For example, $\frac{2}{6} + \frac{5}{6} = \frac{7}{6}$.

5. Describe the process for subtracting fractions with like denominators.

ANSWER: When two fractions have like denominators, you can subtract them by subtracting the top numbers and putting their difference over the denominator. For example, $\frac{4}{8} - \frac{1}{8} = \frac{3}{8}$.

6. Describe the process for adding fractions with unlike denominators.

ANSWER: To add fractions with unlike denominators, you need to find the least common multiple (LCM), which is the smallest answer in a set of multiples that two denominators share in common. For example: $\frac{5}{8} + \frac{6}{16} = \frac{16}{16}$ (or 1).

7. Describe the process for subtracting fractions with unlike denominators.

ANSWER: To subtract fractions with unlike denominators, you need to find the least common multiple (LCM) which is the smallest answer in a set of multiples that two denominators share in common. For example: $\frac{3}{4} - \frac{1}{12} = \frac{8}{12}$

8. Define the greatest common factor method and explain how it is used in multiplying and dividing fractions.

ANSWER: The greatest common factor method is a way of simplifying a fraction by finding the common factors or multipliers of two numbers. It is used in multiplying and dividing fractions that do not have like dominators.

9. What is the cross-canceling method, and how is it used in multiplying fractions?

ANSWER: Cross-canceling occurs when a numerator and a denominator cancel each other out through division by a common factor. Cross-canceling is a simplifying process. We get to the reduced answer more easily by reducing these numbers *before* we multiply.

10. Describe how to divide fractions without using the cross-canceling method.

ANSWER: In order to divide fractions, we must remember this very important rule of thumb: We *never* divide fractions. Instead, we must change the division problem into a multiplication problem. And always change the last fraction to its reciprocal.

11. Explain how to divide fractions using the cross-canceling method.

ANSWER: Remember that cross-canceling is when a numerator and a denominator cancel each other out through division by a common factor. Change the operation from division to multiplication and change the fraction following the operation to its reciprocal.

Let Me Try

LET ME TRY 3–1

Simplify the following fractions.

1. $\dfrac{8}{20} = \dfrac{2}{5}$

2. $\dfrac{15}{35} = \dfrac{3}{7}$

3. $\dfrac{21}{28} = \dfrac{3}{4}$

Find equivalent fractions for the following fractions.

4. $\dfrac{1}{2} = \dfrac{2}{4}, \dfrac{3}{6}, \dfrac{4}{8}, \dfrac{5}{10}$, etc.

5. $\dfrac{3}{5} = \dfrac{6}{10}, \dfrac{9}{15}, \dfrac{12}{20}$, etc.

6. $\dfrac{2}{7} = \dfrac{4}{14}, \dfrac{6}{21}, \dfrac{8}{28}$, etc.

LET ME TRY 3–2

1. $\dfrac{3}{5} + \dfrac{2}{5} = \dfrac{5}{5}$ or **1**

2. $\dfrac{6}{11} - \dfrac{5}{11} = \dfrac{1}{11}$

3. $\dfrac{3}{5} + \dfrac{1}{3} = \dfrac{14}{15}$

4. $\dfrac{5}{6} - \dfrac{3}{4} = \dfrac{1}{12}$

LET ME TRY 3–3

1. $\dfrac{1}{2} \times \dfrac{3}{4} = \dfrac{3}{8}$

2. $\dfrac{3}{7} \times \dfrac{5}{8} = \dfrac{15}{56}$

3. $\dfrac{5}{7} \times \dfrac{3}{5} = \dfrac{3}{7}$

4. $\dfrac{16}{35} \times \dfrac{7}{8} = \dfrac{2}{5}$

LET ME TRY 3–4

1. $\dfrac{3}{7} \div \dfrac{4}{7} = \dfrac{3}{4}$

2. $\dfrac{5}{8} \div \dfrac{15}{40} = \dfrac{5}{3}$

3. $\dfrac{21}{25} \div \dfrac{14}{15} = \dfrac{9}{10}$

4. $\dfrac{32}{45} \div \dfrac{24}{30} = \dfrac{8}{9}$

CHAPTER 4
Review Questions

1. What is a decimal and what does it look like?
ANSWER: Decimals are like fractions because they represent a piece or a part of a whole number. Decimals are numbers to the right or left of a decimal point. The numbers to the right of the decimal represent a piece or a part of a whole dollar. All decimals have equivalent fraction and percent values. An example of a decimal is .75.

2. Add 534.87 and 45.09.
ANSWER: $534.87 + 45.09 = 579.96$

3. Subtract 34.76 from 100.43.
ANSWER: $100.43 - 34.76 = 65.67$

4. Multiply 32.12 by 18.
ANSWER: $32.12 \times 18 = 578.16$

5. Divide 564.98 by 98.36.
ANSWER: $564.98 \div 98.36 = 5.74$

6. Convert the fraction $\dfrac{5}{21}$ to a decimal.
ANSWER: $5 \div 21 = .2380952$

7. Convert the decimal .643 to a percentage.
ANSWER: $.643 = 64\%$

8. Define exponents and explain how they are used.
ANSWER: Exponents are special types of multiplication problems whereby the same number is multiplied by itself as many times as stated by the power. Exponents are used to simplify multiplication problems.

9. Give three examples of exponents, and write a mathematical equation that explains each.
ANSWER: Three examples of exponents and the mathematical equation that explains each are as follows:
3^4 means $3 \times 3 \times 3 \times 3 = 81$
6^3 means $6 \times 6 \times 6 = 216$
8^9 means $8 \times 8 \times 8 \times 8 \times 8 \times 8 \times 8 \times 8 \times 8 = 134{,}217{,}728$

10. Multiply the following exponents: 6^9, 12^3, 3^6.
ANSWER:
$6^9 = 10{,}077{,}696$
$12^3 = 1{,}728$
$3^6 = 729$

11. What is PEMDAS and what does it stand for?
ANSWER: PEMDAS is an acronym that was created by taking the first letter of each of the operations in the order in which they should be done. PEMDAS stands for: **P:** Parentheses; **E:** Exponents; **M:** Multiplication; **D:** Division; **A:** Addition; and **S:** Subtraction.

Let Me Try

1. What is the place value of the digit 7 in the number 173.456?
ANSWER: Tens

2. What is the place value of the digit 6 in the number 183.256?
ANSWER: Thousandths

3. What is the place value of the digit 9 in the number .00295?
ANSWER: Ten thousandths

LET ME TRY 4–2

1. $215.35 + 165 = \mathbf{380.35}$
2. $34.24 + 12.7 = \mathbf{46.94}$
3. $15 + 46.38 = \mathbf{61.38}$
4. $35.67 - 22.89 = \mathbf{12.78}$
5. $16 - 12.67 = \mathbf{3.33}$
6. $214.68 - 178.59 = \mathbf{36.09}$

LET ME TRY 4–3

1. $32.56 \times 12 = \mathbf{390.72}$
2. $23.45 \times 3.45 = \mathbf{80.9025}$
3. $2.345 \times 100 = \mathbf{234.5}$
4. $61.52 \div 15.38 = \mathbf{4}$
5. $12.36 \div .02 = \mathbf{618}$
6. $512.6 \div 2.13 = \mathbf{240.657277}$

LET ME TRY 4–4

For the following equations, give the exponential form of the problem.
1. $5 \times 5 \times 5 \times 5 \times 5 \times 5 \times 5 = \mathbf{5^7}$
2. $3 \times 3 \times 3 \times 3 = \mathbf{3^4}$
3. $6 \times 6 = \mathbf{6^2}$
For the following equations, give the standard form of the problem.
4. $2^4 = \mathbf{2 \times 2 \times 2 \times 2}$
5. $8^2 = \mathbf{8 \times 8}$
6. $3^2 \times 3^3 = \mathbf{3 \times 3 \times 3 \times 3 \times 3}$

LET ME TRY 4–5

Solve these problems. Remember to follow the correct order of operations.
1. $4 \times 3^2 - 3 = \mathbf{33}$
2. $(10 + 20) \div 5 = \mathbf{6}$
3. $10 + (20 \div 5) = \mathbf{14}$
4. $8 \times 3 + 2 \times 5 = \mathbf{34}$
5. $5 + (2 \times 2 + 4)^2 = \mathbf{69}$
6. $5 \times (3^2 - 7) = \mathbf{10}$

CHAPTER 5
Review Questions

1. What is a promotion? Why and when are promotions used in the salon and spa business?
ANSWER: A promotion is a campaign or special that promotes the furtherance of the acceptance and sale of merchandise through advertising, publicity, or discounting to get more clients into the business. Promotions are used to increase business, traffic to the salon, and sales of retail and services.

2. Describe the standard product pricing strategy used in the salon and spa business. If products are purchased at the prices of $4.39, $2.98, $11.76, and $1.86, what would their sales price be?
ANSWER: Most salons and spas double their purchase price to create their sales price, rounding up to the nearest figure. For a product that costs the salon $4.39, its sales price would be $9.00, a product costing $2.98 would be sold for $6.00, a product costing $11.76 would be sold for $24.00, and a product costing $1.86 would be sold for $4.00.

3. Describe the standard service pricing strategy used in the salon and spa business, and name the costs that help determine the final price of a service.
ANSWER: The standard service pricing strategy used in the salon and spa business is to add up all of the costs of performing the service and then to add 30% to 50% on top of those costs to determine the final service price. The costs associated with services offered refer to products used in the performance of the service, supplies used in the performance of the service, overhead, employee commission or salary for performing the service, and any proposed discount or promotion.

4. What is a target profit margin, and how is it helpful when determining pricing and promotions?
ANSWER: The target profit margin is a bare minimum amount of profit that must be made on every sale of product or service, below which it becomes impossible or is no longer desirable to provide services and treatments. Knowing the target profit margin is important to know before planning a promotion, sale, or discount program so that these do not significantly eat into salon profits.

5. Define and describe profit.
ANSWER: Profit is the excess of the selling price of goods after their cost has been subtracted and can be defined further in two ways—as gross profit and net profit. *Gross profit* is simply the difference between sales and costs of sales, meaning product usage. *Net profit* is the revenue left over after the cost of the service (products used) and expenses (such as overhead, advertising, etc.) are subtracted from the sales.

6. What is the Formula Table and how is it used?
ANSWER: The Formula Table is an easy reference for determining how to solve everyday business problems, such as determining taxes, discounts, and sales price.

7. Write a mathematical expression that best describes the following: Heather sells pumice stones for $4.85 each and the sales tax is 7%. What is the sales price of each pumice stone, including the sales tax?
ANSWER: $4.85 \times .07 = .3395$ or .34 (tax to be added to sales price)
$4.85 + .34 = $5.19
The sales price for each pumice stone including the sales tax is $5.19.

8. Simplify this mathematical expression: $(3x + 5) + (2x + 7)$.
ANSWER:
$3x + 5 + 2x + 7 =$
$3x + 2x = 5x$ and $5 + 7 = 12$
therefore $(3x + 5) + (2x + 7) = 5x + 12$

Let Me Try

1. Marie purchased an unknown number of bottles of cuticle softener for $5 per bottle and sold them for $8 per bottle. What mathematic expression represents Marie's total profit?

ANSWER: $8x - 5x$

2. Frank purchased 7 jars of styling wax and 4 cans of hairspray for the same price. What mathematic expression represents Frank's total cost?

ANSWER: $7x + 4x$

3. David sold an unknown number of bottles of top coat on Monday, and on Tuesday he sold 8 more bottles of top coat for $5 per bottle. David paid $33 for all of the bottles. What mathematical expression represents David's total profit?

ANSWER: $5(x + 8) - 33$

1. Jack purchased 6 bottles of nail polish for $3 each.

    a. What formula represents Jack's cost?

    ANSWER: Cost = Price × Quantity

    b. Evaluate the formula if $Q = 6$, $P = \$3$

    ANSWER: Cost = 3 × 6

    c. What is Jack's cost for the 6 bottles of nail polish?

    ANSWER: $18

2. Janice charges $75 for a full set of gel nails but decides to give a 20% discount to attract new customers.

    a. What formula represents the sale price?

    ANSWER: Sales price = price – discount + taxes

    b. If no tax is charged on the service, what is the formula?

    ANSWER: Sales price = price – discount

    c. Evaluate the formula if $P = \$75$, and $R = .20$.

    ANSWER: $S = 75 - (75 \times .20)$

    d. What is the discounted price for the service?

    ANSWER: $S = 75 - (15) = \$60$

3. Annie sells a bottle of hand lotion for $5.69 plus sales tax, which is 7%.

    a. What formula represents the sales price?

    ANSWER: Sales price = price – discount + taxes

    b. The bottle of hand lotion is sold at full price, with no discounts, what formula now represents the same price?

    ANSWER: Sales price = (price × rate)

    c. Evaluate the formula if $P = \$5.69$ and $R = .07$.

    ANSWER: $S = 5.69 + (5.69 \times .07)$, $S = 5.69 + (.40)$ rounded to the nearest penny

    d. What is the price for the bottle of hand lotion?

    ANSWER: $S = \$6.09$

4. Marshall decides to run a special on pedicures. Marshall's spa normally charges $65 for a pedicure, but for the next week, he decides to offer a 15% discount to attract new customers.

    a. What formula represents the net profit for this promotion?

    ANSWER: $N = S - (C + E)$

b. What is the sale price of the pedicure?
ANSWER: $S = P - D, S = 65 - .15$ or $S = \$55.25$

c. Now assume that the costs and expenses involved in giving a pedicure are: $1.50 for service products; $.50 for the clean linens used during the service; $27.62 representing a 50% commission to the pedicurist; $.76 for the cost of advertising the special; and finally $3.25 for overhead, rent, electrical, etc. What is the total cost to the salon of offering this pedicure promotion?
ANSWER: Total cost = $1.5 + $.50 + $27.62 + $.76 + $3.25 = $33.63

d. What is the net profit per pedicure that the salon will see once the pedicure promotion is underway?
ANSWER: $N = \$55.25 - (\$33.63)$, or $21.62.

CHAPTER 6
Review Questions

1. What is an equation and how is it used in calculating profits?
ANSWER: Equations are mathematic statements that define two expressions as being equal to each other, such as in this example: $5 + $5 + $5 + $5 = $20. We work with equations to find a solution, a numerical value that can replace a variable and cause the equation to be true. In other words, the right side will be equal to the left side after all of the operations are performed.

2. Define an algorithm and name the three types used in solving equations.
ANSWER: An algorithm is a mathematical process that is used to arrive at a desired outcome or solution. Three types of algorithms used in solving equations are 1) The Trial and Error Method, 2) The Addition Method, and 3) The Multiplication Method.

3. What is the trial and error method of solving an equation?
ANSWER: The trial and error method is an algorithm that requires the replacement of the variable with an estimated value until the correct value is found. The idea is to try to solve the equation with a new number each time until the correct value is found. Trial and error is a *guess and prove* method.

4. Define the addition method of solving an equation and explain when it is used.
ANSWER: The addition method is an algorithm that requires the use of addition and subtraction to eliminate all values near the variable until the variable is isolated. The addition method is used when the equation involves addition or subtraction.

5. Define the multiplication method of solving an equation and explain when it is used.
ANSWER: The multiplication method is an algorithm that requires the use of multiplication and division to eliminate all values near the variable until the variable is isolated. The multiplication method is used when the equation involves multiplication or division.

Let Me Try

LET ME TRY 6–1
1. Fefe charges $25 per manicure and paid a total of $10 for all her supplies. After subtracting the cost of supplies, she earned $65 on Tuesday.
   a. What equation represents Fefe's profit?
   ANSWER: $\$25x - \$10 = \$65$

   b. Utilizing the trial and error method, how many manicures did Fefe sell?
   ANSWER: 3

2. Cheryl purchased 4 cans of finishing spray for $6 each. She wants to make a total profit of $36 from the sale of all 4 bottles.

  a. What equation represents Cheryl's gross profit?
  ANSWER: $4x - \$24 = \$36$

  b. Utilizing the addition and multiplication methods, what was Cheryl's sales price per bottle?
  ANSWER: $15

3. Martine charges $60 for a full-head haircolor service and made a total of $540 from the sale of haircolor services for the week.

  a. What equation represents Martine's total haircolor sales?
  ANSWER: $\$60x = \$540$

  b. Utilizing the multiplication method, how many haircolor services did Martine perform?
  ANSWER: 9

4. Tishla is trying to determine how many regular and how many spa pedicures she has to sell to earn the same amount of money. Tishla charges $30 for a regular pedicure, and her total supply cost is $18; she charges $40 for a spa pedicure, and her total supply cost is $78.

  a. What equation represents Tishla's situation?
  ANSWER: $\$30x - \$18 = \$40x - \$78$

  b. How many pedicures does Tishla need to sell of each?
  ANSWER: 6

LET ME TRY 6–2

Lonnie has $40 to purchase two different types of shampoo. Shampoo "x" costs $5 per bottle and shampoo "y" costs $8 per bottle. How many bottles of each type of shampoo can Lonnie purchase?

  a. Write an equation that represents the problem.
  ANSWER: $5x + 8y = 40$

  b. How many bottles of each type of shampoo can Lonnie purchase? Give at least 3 solutions.
  ANSWER: Multiple solutions: for example, if $x = 2$, then $y = 3$; if $x = 3$, then $y = 3$; if $x = 4$, then $y = 2$.

CHAPTER 7
Review Questions

1. How are graphs used in business reporting, and what do they allow you to see?
ANSWER: A graph is a mathematical picture that expresses or defines a solution to a problem. A graph is a picture that allows us to compare and establish patterns regarding numbers and outcomes. This is very important because it allows us to see what has occurred over an extended period of time and allows us to use that past history to make predictions about what is likely to happen in the future.

2. Define correlations. Why are they important in business reporting?
ANSWER: A correlation is a relationship between two things. In graphing it is the relationship between the numbers represented both vertically and horizontally on the graph. The correlation is a pattern that allows the reader to observe the past and make predictions about the future based upon the past.

3. What information is found on an income statement? What information is found on a balance sheet?
ANSWER: An *income statement* is a financial report that contains information on the company's income, expense, and net profit. A *balance sheet* is a financial report that contains information on the company's assets, liabilities, and equity.

4. What is the difference between revenue and expense?

ANSWER: The difference between revenue and expense is that *revenue* is the income that a company generates through sales from services and products, while *expense* is the cost or bills that a company pays such as rent, utilities, supplies, telephone, advertising, etc.

5. Describe how to determine percentage of revenue for each service offered in a salon or spa.

ANSWER: To determine percentage of revenue for each service offered in a salon or spa, you would divide the service revenue by the total service revenue. For example, if Body Treatments totaled $67,600 and the total salon revenue totaled $125,000, you would divide $67,600 by $125,000 which equals .5408, or 54%.

6. Describe the type of graph that allows you to compare and contrast figures from current and past financial statements.

ANSWER: A bar graph is used to compare and contrast revenue. The information from the income statement is be used to complete the graph.

7. Explain the difference between variable and fixed costs, and give examples of each.

ANSWER: *Variable costs* are costs that are directly linked to the ability to service a client and will increase or decrease as the number of clients increases or decreases. Examples of variable costs are tubes of haircolor, bottles of shampoo, and clean capes. *Fixed costs* are costs or expenses that never or rarely change. Fixed costs may include: rent, utilities, licenses, fees, tax, telephone, and depreciation.

8. What is a business's break-even point?

ANSWER: A business's break-even point is an equation that defines a point where the revenue and cost are the same, or even.

Let Me Try

LET ME TRY 7–1

1. Jonathon decides to create a pie graph to compare and contrast expenses. Please use the information from his income statement to complete the table below. All decimals will be rounded to the nearest hundredth of a decimal.

Source of Expenses	Identify the Ratios	Convert to a Decimal	Convert to a Percent
1. Rent	$24,000 / $71,680	.34	34%
2. Utilities	$1,800 / $71,680	.03	3%
3. Taxes & Licenses	$2,100 / $71,680	.03	3%
4. Depreciation	$1,600 / $71,680	.02	2%
5. Supplies (service related)	$15,300 / $71,680	.21	21%
6. Travel	$1,600 / $71,680	.02	2%
7. Office Supplies	$1,350 / $71,680	.02	2%
8. Telephone	$960 / $71,680	.01	1%
9. Advertising	$4,250 / $71,680	.06	6%
10. Labor	$18,720 / $71,680	.26	26%
Expenses	$71,680 / $71,680	1.00	100%

© Milady, a part of Cengage Learning.

Now that you have completed filling in the information in the table above, which of the following graphs represents the expenses of Jonathon's Day Spa: Graph A or Graph B?

ANSWER: Graph A correctly represents the expenses of Jonathon's Day Spa. This is the correct graph because the pie chart allocations match the percentages listed on Johnathon's income statement.

Expenses

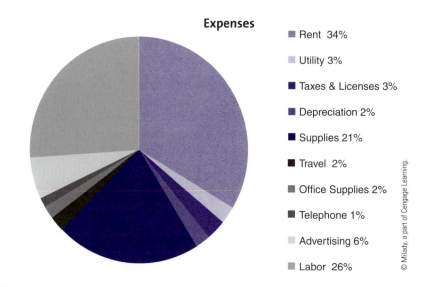

- ■ Rent 34%
- ■ Utility 3%
- ■ Taxes & Licenses 3%
- ■ Depreciation 2%
- ■ Supplies 21%
- ■ Travel 2%
- ■ Office Supplies 2%
- ■ Telephone 1%
- ■ Advertising 6%
- ■ Labor 26%

© Milady, a part of Cengage Learning.

2. Jonathon decides to create a bar graph to compare and contrast expenses. Please use the information from his income statement to complete the problem.

Source of Expenses	Amounts
1. Rent	$24,000
2. Utilities	$1,800
3. Taxes & Licenses	$2,100
4. Depreciation	$1,600
5. Supplies (service related)	$15,300
6. Travel	$1,600
7. Office Supplies	$1,350
8. Telephone	$960
9. Advertising	$4,250
10. Labor	$18,720
Total Expenses	$71,680

© Milady, a part of Cengage Learning.

Which bar graph below represents the expenses of Jonathon's Day Spa: Graph A or Graph B?

ANSWER: Graph A more accurately represents the expenses of Jonathon's Day Spa. This is the correct graph because the height of the bars in the chart matches the expenses of Johnathon's Day Spa.

Graph A

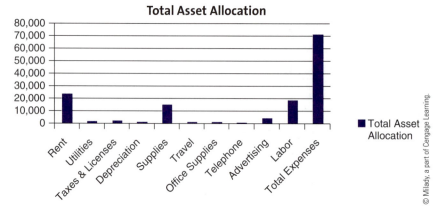

© Milady, a part of Cengage Learning.

3. Jonathon decides to create a line graph to compare and contrast net profit from the current and prior years. Please use the information below to create the line graph.

Net Profit	
2012	$49,750
2011	$61,300
2010	$40,675
2009	$46,232
2008	$43,128

© Milady, a part of Cengage Learning.

ANSWER:

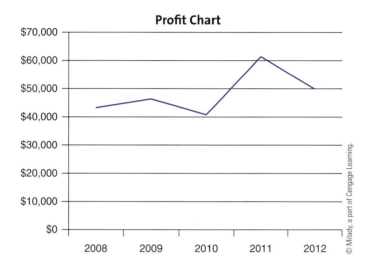

© Milady, a part of Cengage Learning.

LET ME TRY 7–2

1. Create a graph to get a better understanding of Jonathon's ability to generate revenue in 2011 based upon his 2010 total revenue. Jonathon's 2010 revenue consisted of Body Treatments of $55,000; Facials of $36,000; Massage of $27,000; and Retail Sales of $22,000. Jonathon's appointment book indicates that his day spa serviced 2,000 clients in 2010.

ANSWER:

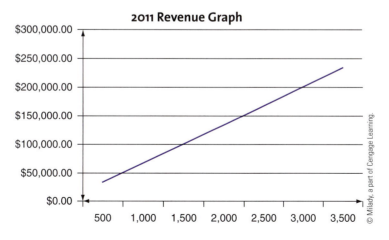

© Milady, a part of Cengage Learning.

2. Create a graph to get a better understanding of Jonathon's total cost in 2011 based upon his total cost in 2010. Jonathon's fixed costs for the prior year, 2010, consisted of: Rent of $22,000; Utilities of $1,900; Taxes/Licenses of $2,000; Depreciation of $1,600, Telephone of $1,000; and Advertising of $3,900. Jonathon's variable cost for the prior year, 2010, consisted of: Products/Supplies $20,400; Office Supplies $1,600; and Labor $18,000. Jonathon's appointment book indicates that his day spa serviced 2,000 clients in 2010.

Answer:

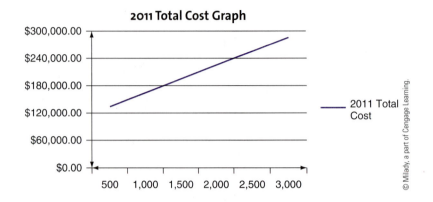

2011 Total Cost Graph

3. Use the information from question 1 and question 2 to find Jonathon's break-even point for 2011.

ANSWER:

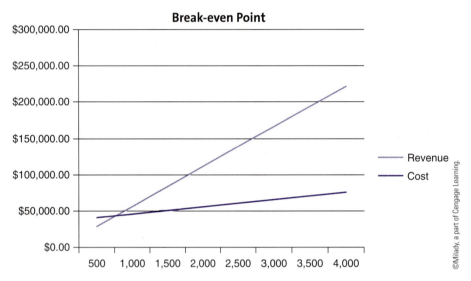

Break-even Point

4. Take a look at the following graph. What information does it indicate to you?

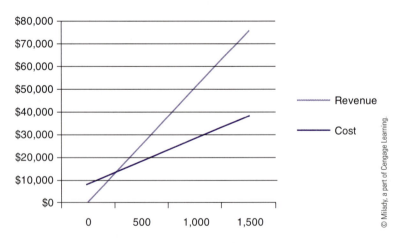

ANSWER:
   a. Revenues were approximately $75,000.
   b. Costs were approximately $40,000.
   c. The break-even point for this business is approximately $14,000.

5. Take a look at the following graph. What information does it indicate to you?

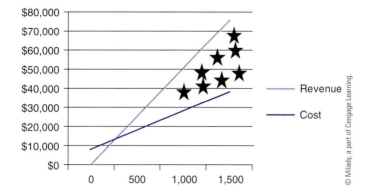

ANSWER:

   a. Revenues were approximately $75,000.
   b. Costs were approximately $40,000.
   c. The break-even point for this business is approximately $14,000.
   d. The stars indicate the possibility for this business to increase its revenue begin at servicing more than approximately 500 clients.

CHAPTER 8
Review Questions

1. Name the two types of measurements systems used today.
ANSWER: The two types of measurements systems used today are the English Measurement System and the Metric System.

2. How does each system measure distance, mass, and volume?
ANSWER: The English Measurement System measures distance by assuming that 12 inches equal 1 foot; 3 feet equals 1 yard; and 1760 yards equal 1 mile. When measuring mass or weight, English Measurement says that 16 ounces equal 1 pound, and 2,000 pounds equal 1 ton. In the case of volume or measuring liquid, 8 ounces equal 1 cup; 2 cups equal 1 pint; 2 pints equal 1 quart; and 4 quarts equal 1 gallon.

The metric system is a system of measurement that measure solids, liquids, and distance with three basic units. The three basic units are: *grams*, *liters*, and *meters*. The three basic units can be increased or decreased with prefixes.

When measuring distance:

- 1 kilometer equals 1000 meters
- 1 hectometer equals 100 meters
- 1 decameter equals 10 meters
- 10 decimeters equals 1 meter
- 100 centimeters equals 1 meter
- 1000 millimeters equals 1 meter

When measuring mass or weight:

- 1 kilogram equals 1,000 grams
- 1 hectogram equals 100 grams
- 1 decagram equals 10 grams

- Gram
  - ➢ 10 decigrams equal 1 gram
  - ➢ 100 centigrams equals 1 gram
  - ➢ 1,000 milligram equals 1 gram

When measuring volume or liquid:

- 1 kiloliter equals 1,000 liters
- 1 hectoliter equals 100 liters
- 1 decaliter equals 10 liters
  - Liter
    - ➢ 10 deciliters equal 1 liter
    - ➢ 100 centiliters equal 1 liter
    - ➢ 1,000 milliliters equal 1 liter

3. What are the steps involved in converting an English measurement to a metric measurement?
ANSWER: First, determine the rates needed to solve the problem. Second, perform any operations required to simplify the rates. Third, combine the rates and multiply them. Finally, interpret the results and apply logic to the outcome.

4. What are the steps involved in converting a metric measurement to an English measurement?
ANSWER: First, determine the rates needed to solve the problem. Second, cross multiply by multiplying a numerator by a denominator. Third, isolate x and solve the problem. Finally, interpret the results and apply logic to the outcome.

Let Me Try

LET ME TRY 8–1
1. Convert 2.86 decagrams to centigrams.
ANSWER: 2,860 centigrams

2. Convert 36 centiliters to liters.
ANSWER: .36 liter

3. Convert 38 ounces to pints.
ANSWER: 2.37 pints

4. Convert 3.7 gallons to ounces.
ANSWER: 473.6 ounces

5. Convert 3 gallons to liters.
ANSWER: 11.36 liters

6. Convert 823 liters to ounces.
ANSWER: 27,828.94 ounces

CHAPTER 9
Review Questions

1. Define and explain the difference between a beginning balance and an ending balance as indicated on a bank statement.

ANSWER: The beginning balance indicated on a bank statement is the amount of money the account has in it at the start of the period, usually a month. The ending balance is the amount of money the account has in it at the end of the month.

2. What is the difference between principal and interest?
ANSWER: *Principal* is the word used to describe the original monies put into an account. *Interest* is the fee a bank pays for using a customer's money.

Let Me Try

LET ME TRY 9–1
1. If a bank account has a beginning balance of $8,137.43, deposits of $10,346.31, checks of $6,531.21, bank charges of $39.86, and withdrawals of $561.39, how much is the ending balance?
ANSWER: $11,351.28

2. If a bank account has a beginning balance of $19,749.41, checks of $10,563.83, bank charges of $41.37, other credits of $33.67, and an ending balance of $21,894.79, how much are the deposits?
ANSWER: $12,716.91

3. Use the following information to find the annual interest rate.
Interest paid (i) = $500
Principal (p) = $8,000
Rate (r) = ?
ANSWER: 6.25%

4. Use the following information to find the simple interest rate.
Principal (p) = $10,000
Annual interest rate (r) = 7.25%
Time (t) = 5 years
Interest paid (i) = ?
ANSWER: $3,625

5. Use the following information to find the future value of simple interest.
Future value (Fv) = ?
Principal (p) = $5,000
Annual interest rate (r) = 6%
Time (t) = 10 years
ANSWER: $8,000

CHAPTER 10
Review Questions

1. What is inventory, and why is it useful to track it carefully?
ANSWER: Inventory is a collection of supplies and products that a company uses to generate sales. It is useful to track it carefully so you can always know how much merchandise you have on hand, can plan for special sales promotions that may cause sales to increase, and so that you can track any loss of inventory which costs the salon or spa additional monies.

2. Define periodic and perpetual inventory systems, and describe which types of products in a salon or spa may be tracked by each method.

ANSWER: A *periodic* inventory system is tracked by counting the inventory daily, weekly, or monthly. The types of products you would track with this system include backbar and service/treatment products. A *perpetual* inventory system is tracked administratively through purchase orders, sales invoices, and counting the inventory quarterly, semiannually, or annually. Perpetual inventory is how salons and spas account for products that they purchase in bulk, such as gallons of massage oil, cleansers, shampoos or conditioners, and how they inventory their retail-size products for sale to clients.

3. What is an item's unit price and how is it determined?

ANSWER: The unit price of an item is the amount that is paid for each individual unit. The formula for determining unit price is Unit Price $= \frac{Total\ Price}{Total\ Units}$.

4. How is time defined? Name the four types of time that are tracked in a business setting.

ANSWER: Time is defined as a quantitative measurement that accounts for the initiation and expiration of all things. The four types of time tracked in a business setting are idle time, administrative time, work time, and overlapping time.

5. What are the general steps involved in converting time from one form of measurement to another form of measurement?

ANSWER: We can convert time by changing one measurement of time to another measurement of time so that it can be added or subtracted. Typically, time is converted from a larger unit to a smaller unit of measurement.

6. On Tuesday John is booked for 1 hour on a haircolor, $1\frac{1}{2}$ hours styling an updo, and 45 minutes on a haircut. How long will John spend in the salon on Tuesday?

ANSWER: John will spend 3 hours and 15 minutes in the salon on Tuesday.

7. Andy has a doctor's appointment on Friday and plans on using 4 personal hours so he can go to the doctor. If he usually works 5 days in the salon, how many days will Andy work that week?

ANSWER: Andy will work 5 days in the salon: 4 full days and 1 half day.

8. Bonnie has 2 hours open on Saturday, when a client calls to book two facials for that same day. Each facial is 75 minutes long. Can Bonnie accommodate the request?

ANSWER: Bonnie can accommodate one client for one facial on Saturday. She has 120 minutes free, but two facials will require 150 minutes.

9. Amy has 3 free hours and donates that time to a shelter for homeless children. It takes her 40 minutes to complete 1 haircut, so how many haircuts can she perform in 3 hours during her time at the homeless shelter?

ANSWER: Amy can comfortably perform 4 haircuts in a 3-hour window of time.

Let Me Try

LET ME TRY 10–1

1. Use the information below to determine how much shampoo, conditioner, and 3-ounce tubes of haircolor were used.

Description	Beginning	Purchased	Used	Ending
Shampoo	4 gallons	3 gallons	_____	1 gallon
Conditioner	6 gallons	3 gallons	_____	4 gallons
Haircolor	6 @ 3 ounces	2 @ 3 ounces	_____	4 @ 3 ounces

ANSWER: 6 gallons of shampoo were used; 5 gallons of conditioner were used; 4 tubes of 3-ounce haircolor were used.

2. Use the information below to determine how much shampoo, conditioner, and 3-ounce tubes of haircolor should be left at the end of the month.

Description	Beginning	Purchased	Used	Ending
Shampoo	4 gallons	6 gallons	5 gallons	_____
Conditioner	3 gallons	5 gallons	6 gallons	_____
Haircolor	5 @ 3 ounces	4 @ 3 ounces	6 @ 3 ounces	_____

© Milady, a part of Cengage Learning.

ANSWER: 5 gallons of shampoo, 2 gallons of conditioner, and 3 tubes of 3-ounce haircolor should be left at the end of the month.

3. How many seconds are there in 7.5 hours?
ANSWER: 27,000 seconds

4. How many hours are there in 480 minutes?
ANSWER: 8 hours

5. How many weeks are in 154 days?
ANSWER: 22 weeks

6. If Arlene's calendar shows that she has 1 haircolor scheduled today, which will take 75 minutes, and 5 perms scheduled at 2.25 hours for each, at what time will Arlene finish if she starts at 8 a.m.?
ANSWER: Arlene will finish work at approximately 9:30 p.m. if she works straight through the day without any breaks.

7. If David performed 6 haircuts with an average time of 25 minutes each, 8 shaves with an average time of 30 minutes each, and 3 perms with an average time of 2¼ hours each, how many hours did he spend all together on the haircuts, shaves, and perms?
ANSWER: David spent 13 hours and 15 minutes performing all of this work.

Glossary

A

absolute value bars—Grouping symbols that measure a number's distance from zero.

addends—The numbers that are being added together.

addition—The combining of two or more groups of the same objects.

addition method—An algorithm that requires the use of addition and subtraction to eliminate all values near the variable until the variable is isolated. The addition method is used when the equation involves addition or subtraction.

administrative time—Also known as *indirect labor*; the time spent doing paperwork and making decisions.

algorithm—A mathematical process that is used to arrive at a desired outcome or solution.

amortization of a simple loan—The process of repaying a loan with equal periodic payments.

annual interest rate—The ratio of interest to principal before compounding any interest.

assets—Items that a company owns that can generate money or be converted into money, which can include equipment, supplies, money, land, and buildings.

associative property—A property that is used with addition or multiplication, but not both at the same time. The property states that the grouping of the numbers in an equation in different arrangements will not affect the answer.

B

balance sheet—A financial report that compares a company's assets, liabilities and equity.

bar graph—A graph that uses rectangular shapes to compare and contrast numerical values.

base—In relation to exponents, the number that is to be multiplied.

beginning balance—The amount of money the account has in it at the start of the period, usually a month.

boundary—A restriction on the solution that does not allow the solution to extend or go beyond a certain point called the *upper* or *lower limit* of the solution.

brackets—Grouping symbols, similar to parentheses, that allow the grouping of things that are alike or similar to each other together so that they can be combined into one value prior to performing any other operations.

break-even point—An equation that defines a point where the revenue and cost are the same, or even.

C

commutative property—Property that is used with addition or multiplication, but not both at the same time. The commutative property states that moving the numbers around, or changing the order of the numbers, will not affect the answer.

composite number—A number that is divisible by more than 1 and itself.

compound period—The amount of time it takes for interest paid on an account, which then becomes part of the principal and starts earning interest.

compounded interest—The amount of money earned annually from principal or a loan and any past interest.

compounding—The addition of interest to the principal.

constant—A numerical value that is fixed and does not change.

conversion rate—A rate that compares two measurements through division, with the intention of converting one measurement to another measurement.

converting—When the appearance of a number is changed so that the number looks different but still has the same value.

converting multiple rates—A rate that compares three or more measurements through division and multiplication, with the intention of converting measurements to another measurement.

converting time—A process by which one measurement of time is changed to another measurement of time.

correlation—A relationship between two things, such as the numbers represented vertically and the numbers represented horizontally on a graph. The correlation is a pattern that allows the reader to observe the past and make predictions about the future based upon the past.

creditors—The people to whom the money is owed; creditors have rights to the assets of a company if the company cannot pay its debts.

cross-canceling—Cross-canceling is a simplifying process; we can save time and work by using the cross-canceling method when multiplying fractions.

cross multiplication—A mathematical process that is used to compare two equivalent fractions when one of the fractions has an unknown value.

D

decimals—Like fractions because they represent a piece, or a part, of a whole number.

denominator—The bottom number of a fraction.

difference—The answer that the minuend and the subtrahend create.

digits—The numerical symbols that make up a number.

distributive property—A property that is used with multiplication, addition, and subtraction. Multiplication and at least one of the other operations must be present. The distributive property states that we multiply the number on the outside of the parentheses by everything that is on the inside of the parentheses, completing the operation inside the parentheses first.

dividend—The number that is being divided.

division—The reducing of one or more sets of numbers.

divisor—The number that is doing the dividing.

E

effective interest rate—The ratio of interest to principal *after* compounding interest.

ending balance—The amount of money an account has in it at the end of the month.

English measurement—A system of measurements that measures solids, liquids, and distance with different measurement units depending on the quantity and type of item.

equation—A math statement that defines two math expressions as being equal to each other, such as $3x + 7 = 2x - 5$. Also the format mathematics uses to communicate its meaning; for example, $4 + 3 = 7$ is an equation.

equations—Mathematical statements that define two expressions as being equal to each other, such as in this example: $\$5 + \$5 + \$5 + \$5 = \$20$.

equivalent fraction—When two fractions look different but have the same value and are obtained when we either multiply or divide the numerator and the denominator of a fraction by the same number.

evaluating—Replacing variables with some known numerical values and then performing the order of operations.

expense—The cost or bills that a company pays such as rent, utilities, supplies, telephone, advertising, etc.

exponential form—When a problem is written as an exponent, for example, 3^3.

exponents—Special types of multiplication problems whereby the same number is multiplied by itself as many times as stated by the power.

F

factor—A number that can divide into another number and create an answer that is a whole number without a remainder.

factors—The numbers that are being multiplied.

first rule—States that anytime we raise a base to the first power, the answer is the base. For example, $7^1 = 7$.

fixed costs—Costs or expenses that never or rarely change. Fixed costs may include rent, utilities, licenses, fees, tax, telephone, and depreciation.

formula—Also known as a *math expression*; a formula is a math statement that defines a real-world problem in math terms.

fraction—A ratio (the relationship in quantity, amount, or size between two or more things) that compares two numbers by dividing one into the other.

fraction—Counts a portion or piece of something; a ratio that compares two numbers by division.

future value of compound interest—The value that money will be worth in the future, provided it is earning a specific compound interest rate.

future value of simple interest—The value that money will be worth in the future, provided it is earning a specific, non-compound interest rate.

G

graph—A mathematical picture that expresses or defines a solution to a problem.

greatest common factor (GCF)—The largest number that we can divide two or more numbers by.

greatest common factor method—A way of simplifying a fraction by finding the common factors or multipliers of two numbers.

gross profit—The difference between sales and costs of sales, meaning product usage.

I

identity property—A property that is used with addition or multiplication. It states that when zero is added to a number or when a number is multiplied by 1, it will not change the original number. The identity number for addition is 1, and 0 is the identity number for multiplication.

idle time—The time spent doing nothing.

income statement—A report that compares the company's income, expense, and net profit.

integers—Positive or negative whole numbers; for example, 1, 2, and 3 are positive numbers and -1, -2, and -3 are negative numbers.

interest—The fee a bank pays for using a customer's money.

inventory—A collection of supplies and products that a company uses to generate sales.

inverse property—A property that is used with addition or multiplication. The inverse property of addition states that any time you add a number to its opposite the answer is zero.

L

least common denominator or multiple (LCM)—The smallest number that two numbers share in common if we are multiplying or counting by both numbers.

liabilities—Also known as *debt*; the amount of money that the company owes for such things as mortgage notes, car loans, revolving lines of credit, notes payable, and accounts payable.

like denominator fractions—When the bottom numbers of the two fractions are the same.

like terms—Terms that have the same variables and powers or exponents, such as $3x$, $5x$, $6x$, and $7x$.

line graph—A graph that uses straight lines to compare and contrast numerical values.

linear equation—An equation for a straight line. A linear equation describes a relationship in which the value of one of the variables depends on the value of the other variable. It usually has a constant and must have simple variables.

linear inequalities—A comparison symbol used when seeking to compare two things in order to come to a conclusion that one side is either equal to, less than, or greater than the other.

M

math expression—Also known as a *formula*; a math statement that is meaningful and has a collection of numbers, variables, signs, and operations, such as $3x + 7$.

mathematical logic—The science of using correct reasoning.

mathematical operations—Tasks that are performed between two or more numbers or groups of numbers.

mathematical properties—The rules or characteristics that will always exist for a particular mathematical operation.

mathematics—A universal language that is expressed with numbers, graphs, shapes, symbols, and signs of operations.

metric measurement—Also known as *the metric system*; a system of measurement that measures solids, liquids, and distance with three basic units. The three basic units are *grams*, *liters*, and *meters*.

minuend—The number that is being reduced by subtraction.

multiplication—The combining of one or more sets of numbers.

multiplication method—An algorithm that requires the use of multiplication and division to eliminate all values near the variable until the variable is isolated. The multiplication method is used when the equation involves multiplication or division.

N

negative numbers—Reside on the left side of zero on a number line and are the opposite of positive numbers.

net profit—The revenue left over after the cost of the service (products used) and expenses (such as overhead, advertising, etc.) are subtracted from the sales; the difference between the revenue and expenses.

numerator—The top number of a fraction.

O

order of operations—States that when there are different operations in a problem, they must be completed in a specific order. The order is parentheses ( ), exponents, multiplication, division, addition, and subtraction.

overlapping time—Time shared between two or more clients, such as completing a haircut while another client's haircolor processes.

owner's equity—The difference between assets and liabilities. The owner has rights to the assets after the creditors have been paid.

P

parentheses—Grouping symbols that allow us to group things that are alike or similar to each other together so that they can be combined into one value prior to performing any other operations.

PEMDAS—An acronym that was created by taking the first letter of each of the operations in the order that they should be done: P = Parentheses, E = Exponents, M = Multiplication, D = Division, A = Addition, and S = Subtraction.

periodic inventory system—Tracked by counting the inventory daily, weekly, or monthly.

perpetual inventory system—Tracked administratively through purchase orders, sales invoices, and by occasionally counting the inventory quarterly, semiannually, or annually.

pie graph—Also known as *pie chart*; a circular graph that uses pie shapes to compare and contrast numerical values.

place value—The value each digit holds in a specific location in reference to the decimal point in a number.

point of origin—Where a measurement begins. Zero is the point of origin for all numbers.

positive numbers—Reside on the right side of zero on a number line and are the opposite of negative numbers.

power—Also known as *superscript*; the number that determines how many times the base of an exponent is to be multiplied by itself.

prime factorization—Multiplying a group of prime numbers together to come up with a product.

prime fraction—Obtained when a fraction cannot be simplified.

prime number—A number that is divisible by only 1 and itself.

principal—The original monies put into the account.

product—The answer that is created by multiplying the factors.

product rule—States that any time we multiply exponents together that have the same base, we simply add the powers together.

profit—The excess of the selling price of goods after their cost has been subtracted.

profit margin—A bare minimum below which, or an extreme limit beyond which, something becomes impossible or is no longer desirable.

promotions—The furtherance of the acceptance and sale of merchandise through advertising, publicity, or discounting.

Q

quotient—The answer that the dividend and divisor create.

R

radical sign—Grouping symbols that determine the root of a number.

rate—Compares two quantities through division. A rate can be written in several forms: whole numbers, fractions, decimals, and percentages.

ratio—A process that compares two quantities by the basic operation of division.

reciprocal—The inverting of a fraction or, in other words, reversing the top and bottom numbers of the fraction.

revenue—The income that a company generates through sales from services and products.

rounded number—An approximate number rather than an exact number.

S

sign—A symbol in front of a number that allows us to know whether the number is negative or positive.

signed number—When a number is positive, indicated by a + (plus) sign, or negative, indicated by a – (minus) sign, thus indicating which side of the number line it resides on. Signed numbers can be fractions and decimals as well as whole numbers.

simple interest—The amount of money earned annually from principal or on a loan without compounding the interest.

simplified fraction—A fraction obtained when the numerator and the denominator of a fraction are divided by the same number.

simplify—A mathematical process that makes a math expression easier to understand or solve through the use of the order of operation (PEMDAS), associative property, commutative property, and distributive property.

solution—A numerical value that can replace a variable and cause the equation to be true.

standard form—When a problem is written in the usual way, for example, $3 \times 3 \times 3$.

subtraction—The reducing of two or more groups of the same objects.

subtrahend—The number that is being subtracted.

sum—The answer created by the addition of addends.

T

term—A number, or the product of a number, and a variable raised to a power, such as 3, 7, $5y$, or $6x$.

time—A quantitative measurement that accounts for the initiation and expiration of all things.

trial and error method—An algorithm that requires the replacement of the variable with an *estimated* value until the correct value is found.

U

unit measurement—A way of defining an item in numerical terms that allows the quantity of the item to be compared to the quantity of another item.

unit price—The amount that is paid for each unit.

unlike denominator fractions—When the bottom numbers of the two fractions are not the same.

unlike terms—Terms that have different variables or powers or exponents, such as 3, $3x$, $3x^2$, $3y$, and so forth.

V

variable—A letter or symbol that represents some unknown numerical value or values, such as x or y.

variable costs—Costs that are directly linked to the ability to service a client and will increase or decrease as the number of clients increases or decreases.

W

work time—Also known as *direct labor*; the time directly related to rendering a service or selling a product to a client.

Z

zero rule—States that anytime we raise a base to the zero power, the answer is 1. For example, $7^0 = 1$.

Index

Note: Information appearing in tables is denoted by *t*.